POSITIVE
DISINTEGRATION

POSITIVE DISINTEGRATION

"Dąbrowski's theory is not only interesting but even exciting in its breadth and depth of its implications. The ubiquity of psychological symptoms has always confounded a simple descriptive psychopathological approach to mental illness. Dąbrowski's theory gives these symptoms a role in normal personality development that is consistent with their broad distribution as shown by epidemiological studies and as felt by those aware of the problems in themselves and in those around them."

~ *Jason Aronson*, Harvard Medical School

MENTAL GROWTH THROUGH POSITIVE DISINTEGRATION

"I consider this to be one of the most important contributions to psychological and psychiatric theory in this whole decade. There is little question in my mind that this book will be read for another decade or two, and very widely. It digs very deep and comes up with extremely important conclusions that will certainly change the course of psychological theorizing and the practice of psychotherapy for some time to come."

~ *Abraham H. Maslow*, Brandeis University

PERSONALITY SHAPING THROUGH POSITIVE DISINTEGRATION

"Dr. Kazimierz Dąbrowski is no ordinary psychiatrist. Although educated as a physician, he has developed a conception of man and his 'existential' vagaries which radically transcends the physical and biological realms; and although later trained in Freudian psychoanalysis, he has a point of view which, instead of denigrating morality and idealism, puts them in a place of supreme importance.

Dr. Dąbrowski has certainly been a pioneer in the development of the kind of psychiatry that is set forth in this book, and he deserves great credit for his originality and courage. But, at the same time there is nothing singular or eccentric about his particular orientation. It is, in fact, part and parcel of a widespread and growing perspective in clinical psychology and psychiatry which can only be described as revolutionary."

~ *O. Hobart Mowrer*, University of Illinois

POSITIVE
DISINTEGRATION

Kazimierz Dąbrowski, M.D., Ph.D.

Foreword by William Tillier, M.Sc.

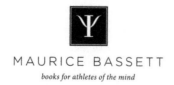

MAURICE BASSETT

books for athletes of the mind

Positive Disintegration

Maurice Bassett
P.O. Box 839
Anna Maria, FL 34216

MauriceBassett@gmail.com
www.MauriceBassett.com

Cover Design by Tammy Arthur
Interior Layout by Chris Nelson

ISBN: 978-1-60025-095-8

Library of Congress Control Number: 2016905070

We wish to thank Bill Tillier for maintaining his promise to keep the theory of positive disintegration alive. Bill has been tenacious and tireless in all his activities related to the theory including, but not limited to, the development of the English website, research, publications, correspondence and active involvement in meetings and conferences. We are especially grateful for Bill's dedication to the word, the intent, the integrity and the soul of the theory.

~ the Dąbrowski family

Contents

Foreword

Positive disintegration. At first glance these two words don't seem to make sense together. How can disintegration—falling apart—be positive?

After studying exemplars of psychological development, Kazimierz Dąbrowski concluded that progressive personality development requires the disintegration of lower integrations of psychological function. When these disintegrations occur they share a common denominator. All involve strong anxiety, self-doubt and depression that challenge the status quo and push the individual to seek more, to try to imagine what could be—what ought to be—in contrast to what is. Dąbrowski concluded that this process is necessary for personal growth and coined the term positive disintegration to describe it.

WHO WAS KAZIMIERZ DĄBROWSKI?

To appreciate how Dąbrowski came to this unusual conclusion it is helpful to understand the personal experiences that shaped his thinking.

Kazimierz Dąbrowski was born in 1902 in Klarów, Poland. As a child, he was profoundly affected by the death of his younger sister and, later, by his experience of walking through the bloody aftermath of a battle near his home during World War I. He was a precocious student, and before obtaining his secondary school certificate he had already passed his first and second year university examinations. During his master's degree studies he considered a career in music, but when his best friend and fellow student committed suicide, Dąbrowski set himself on a path to better understand self-destructive behavior. He studied under some of the most prominent European neurologists, psychologists and psychiatrists of the day. He became a physician, a psychiatrist and a psychologist. During the 1930s, he continued to expand his education, spending a year in America at Harvard University, Johns Hopkins University and at the Boston Psychopathic Hospital. He also began a prolific writing career. With financial support from the Rockefeller Foundation, he established a series of mental health clinics in Poland.

He was ensnared in World War II, narrowly avoiding the concentration camps (he lost two brothers in the war) but nonetheless finding himself imprisoned—first at the hands of the German police and later under Stalin, where he endured eighteen months of torture.

During the 1950s, his activities were closely controlled by the Communist regime, but he continued to push forward his research on self-harm, suicide and personality development. In the 1960s, he was able to establish academic positions in Canada, and published several books in English. He passed away in Poland in 1980, survived by his wife and two daughters.

VAST DIFFERENCES BETWEEN INDIVIDUALS

I was fortunate enough to be Dąbrowski's student in the late 1970s in Edmonton, Alberta. Dąbrowski told me that he first realized there were tremendous differences between individuals when he walked through the field of dead soldiers during World War I. At that time, he was struck by the different expressions frozen on the faces of the men. Some expressed a very calm and serene look, as if they were sleeping. Others showed agony and fear. He explained also that later, in World War II, he witnessed the worst atrocities imaginable but also saw great acts of heroism. After the war he could not find a theory of psychology that could adequately explain these disparate behaviors and the vast continuum of values they must represent.

His observations of people operating at these different levels led him to formalize the theory that two major, qualitatively different types of personality are reflected at the respective poles of a continuum. Dąbrowski also observed and described a process of disintegration involved in personality development. In this context, the process of disintegration is necessary in order to break apart one's lower personality, allowing one to consciously create a higher personality—a process whereby an individual moves from one pole to the other.

TWO TYPES OF PERSONALITY INTEGRATION

Dąbrowski used a conventional approach to integration. Integration reflects a deep unification, organization and coordination of mental functions. A key characteristic of integration is the lack of internal psychological conflicts; the individual is in internal harmony with his or her feelings and behavior, a harmony traditionally associated with normality and mental health.

Dąbrowski outlined two types of personality integration: a lower primary integration—reflecting a **socially-integrated personality**—and the other representing a higher secondary integration—a self-constructed, **autonomous integration**. The basic belief and value systems that are reflected in these two integrations, and more importantly, the source of these beliefs and values, differentiate these integrations.

Primary integration (the socially-integrated personality)

A long tradition in philosophy has described the **socially-integrated personality**, perhaps beginning with Plato's allegory of the cave where so-called prisoners sit passively watching an illusion of life unfold in front of them. The socialized, "average" individual adopts his or her beliefs and values essentially "ready-made" from their social environment—from their parents, peer group and schooling—what Dąbrowski called second-factor influences.

The process of socialization is generally seen to effectively squelch individuality and autonomy; people are molded toward homogeneity, all marching to the same drum.

Few internal psychological conflicts are seen at this level.

The vast majority of conflicts are generated by clashes with the external environment.

Primary integration also includes the antisocial individual who is guided by primitive instincts, ego, selfishness, and hedonism—what Dąbrowski called first-factor influences. These individuals often cannot control their behavior and frequently run afoul of the law, but many also find their way into business or politics, where they tend to excel.

Secondary integration (autonomous integration)

In **autonomous integration**, beliefs and values are consciously chosen based on a deep exploration of one's self. Dąbrowski emphasized the process of self-reflection, self-education, self-directed therapy, and a conscious embracing of higher ideals of life and self and a simultaneous rejection of characteristics perceived to be lower and less congruent with one's basic character. This introspective review leads to the conscious shaping of one's personality toward a unique expression of one's beliefs, values, aims, goals and ideals.

An idealization of one's personality—who one imagines and feels one ought to be—guides one toward secondary integration. This personality ideal creates conflicts and disease when confronted with the status quo of who one is at present. These "is versus ought" conflicts contribute to the motivation to grow and help fuel the disintegrations needed to actively achieve autonomous integration.

Few internal psychological conflicts are seen once full autonomous integration is achieved. This is because one's behavior is congruent with one's values; consequently, moral dilemmas no longer arise. When conflicts *do* arise they are the result of living in an environment at odds with one's own deep values and sensibilities. Secondary (autonomous) integration is rarely seen in practice, but it has been illustrated by many exemplars. These include Abraham Lincoln, Mahatma Gandhi, Helen Keller, Mother Teresa and Martin Luther King, Jr., to name a few.

Dąbrowski emphasized that the individual differences within each type of integration are quantitative, whereas the differences between the two integrations are qualitative; the two integrations are mutually exclusive.

WHY DO SO FEW REACH ADVANCED DEVELOPMENT?

It is generally agreed that very few people realize the highest levels of their potential, however that potential is defined by the different approaches and theories of development. Why should this be the case?

Most theorists conclude that life is simply too harsh and that the wear and tear of everyday living consumes the energy needed for advanced growth.

Dąbrowski said that in order to move to autonomy, the earlier, lower, social integrations must disintegrate. However, primary integration provides compelling security for the individual who follows social roles and "does not step out of the box." There is tremendous rigidity and inertia around engaging in personal development because there is constant social pressure to conform. Conformity generally reduces anxiety. Furthermore, there are, at times, fairly severe consequences for the expression of individuality. As well, Dąbrowski described certain personality traits necessary to overcome this initial integration and, to echo Plato, not everyone is equipped to break free from the cave and make the hard journey into the sunlight.

DEVELOPMENTAL POTENTIAL

Dąbrowski studied exemplars of development and concluded that they all exhibited a combination of personality characteristics that he called developmental potential. This constellation of genetic features determines the type and extent of development possible. These potentials can be negative, equivocal or positive.

Positive developmental potential includes genetic traits reflecting higher, more autonomous and authentic human attributes. These include: developmental instincts, a strong sense of needing to be oneself, special abilities and talents, and over-excitability—to name a few. Over-excitability involves a lowered threshold and a heightened response to the incoming stimuli of the world as compared with the reactions of the "average" individual.

The presence of strong positive developmental potential does not guarantee one will achieve growth, but these factors, in particular a vividness of emotional experience, a strong intellectual curiosity and a vivid imagination, predispose both disintegration and a positive growth outcome for crises and trauma. Strong positive developmental potential can often overcome an ambivalent or negative environment.

If developmental potential is equivocal, then environment becomes a critical determinant. If developmental potential is weak or absent, then advanced development is unlikely, even with a positive environment.

In summary, Dąbrowski believed that the achievement of autonomy required an individual to volitionally inhibit the lower genetic influences that reflect our animal heritage (to consciously resist lower impulses), and to confront and disintegrate socialized, robotic and unreflective behavior. This disintegrative process is not universal for all individuals; it is predicated upon strong developmental potential that both stimulates internal psychological crises and allows an individual to take control of his or her development and create a self-determined personality.

THE HORIZONTAL DILEMMA

Dąbrowski characterized primary (socialized) behavior as unilevel, literally existing on a horizontal plane. Often individuals are faced with a fork in the road: one can turn left or one can turn right. For Dąbrowski, these horizontal, flatland choices are different but essentially equivalent and do not present true opportunities for growth. As long as an individual is locked into this horizontal view, development is thwarted.

Dąbrowski observed that many people show ambivalence over which choice to make. Some also show ambitendencies; that is, they go one way, then change course and go in the other direction. This may develop into a unilevel disintegration—a very stressful process because the individual feels locked into a hopeless situation with no obvious way out. Often the individual in unilevel disintegration regresses back into the stability of primary integration ("don't rock the boat, go with the flow and everything will be okay"). If conditions are optimal, however, the individual may find a developmental solution by pushing forward into further growth and multilevelness.

THE HIERARCHICAL VIEW OF LIFE

The resolution of the horizontal dilemma, and the key to personality development, is the emergence of a hierarchical view of life. In the search for more and better solutions, an individual with a strong imagination can see "the possibility of the higher," and this creates a radically new, vertical perception of reality. Multilevelness allows the individual to rise above the stimulus-response, largely unconscious behavior that characterizes unilevel primary integration. *Left* versus *right* choices yield to the challenge of making lower versus higher decisions. One's options are now evaluated as *lower* or *higher*, especially in the context of one's historical choices. The behavior displayed by others also comes to be judged by this vertical criterion.

When vertical choices confront a person, he or she often initially chooses the lower course. When this happens, the person may experience guilt and remorse. These experiences accumulate and, over time, the higher choices come to be valued and acted on. In synergy with the development of the autonomous integration of personality, multilevelness helps create a new and deeper appreciation of the meaning of life. The theory is not prescriptive: the individual must discover his or her own prioritization of values and ideals.

THE THREE FACTORS

As we have seen, Dąbrowski described first factor influences that reflect the influence of genetic characteristics; here he was primarily concerned with the lower instincts of our primate heritage. The second factor represents environmental and social influences that tend to control and direct behavior and development. Dąbrowski saw that exemplars exhibit a third force—the third factor. The third factor is a strong internal drive that emerges from one's higher genetic traits to motivate one toward the achievement of one's individuality. More than simple willpower, this factor is a drive motivating self-determination and expression.

Given this context we can answer the question: How can we reconcile the vast differences seen in behavior between individuals?

These differences reflect the lower primary integration that includes a small number of antisocial individuals as well as the majority of the socialized population. Criminal behavior, sometimes of horrific magnitude, is commonly associated with antisocial individuals, whereas the average individual generally follows the mores and values of the prevailing society. Here, the average person generally falls in step with these prevailing rules and regulations, but compliance is generally highest when there is a policeman standing on the corner. Often, harsh or unethical behavior is socially justified—for example, in the dog-eat-dog business world.

At the other end of the spectrum are individuals who have achieved a sense of multilevelness and autonomy. With advancing development, it becomes less and less likely that an individual will engage in behaviors that harm others. At the highest levels, self-defined and self-determined individuals will defend their beliefs at all costs, and self-sacrifice to save others is not uncommon. Dąbrowski cited the example of Saint Maximilian Maria Kolbe, a Polish priest who volunteered to take the place of a fellow prisoner slated for death in Auschwitz (the other prisoner, Franciszek Gajowniczek, survived the war, reuniting with his family and living to the age of ninety-three).

In summary, Dąbrowski contended that the broad range of behaviors displayed by people reflect fundamental differences in the personalities and characteristics of the individuals involved.

THREE TYPES OF DISINTEGRATION

Dąbrowski described three types of disintegration. The first is unilevel in nature and is experienced as a short, intense crisis with little hope of solution. An example of this might be an individual who is happily engaged to be married. He or she meets someone new at work and they feel love at first sight. Acting on these emotions, the person finds him or herself in love with two people. Both attractions are strong and one is left to agonize over whom to choose. Eventually circumstances may force one choice or the other and the individual is able to end the crisis, returning to a stable and monogamous relationship.

Two types of multilevel disintegration are differentiated. The first occurs spontaneously, usually in response to external stimuli that one experiences as upsetting. The second occurs when, with further development, disintegrations come to be actively directed by the individual. Lower and undesirable aspects of one's personality are recognized and targeted to be actively dismantled and transformed. In this manner, one inhibits those features perceived as lower and actualizes those features perceived as higher. I have described this process as multilevel actualization. (In describing self-actualization, Maslow did not make this vertical distinction; he advocated the actualization of all potentials, both the lower and higher.)

LOCUS AND NATURE OF CONFLICTS IN DISINTEGRATION

In positive disintegration, conflicts become internalized and usually involve strong anxieties, questioning of oneself, depression and feelings of being lost, inferior and hopeless. Dąbrowski called these psychoneuroses and saw them as a necessary, critical part of the developmental process—there is no potential for growth when homeostasis prevails. In a developmental context, these psychological states provide the dis–ease that motivates one to question one's beliefs and values, to seek new answers, to discover one's deeper self, and to move toward the expression of individuality.

A SUMMARY OF DĄBROWSKI'S LEVELS

The theory is presented as five levels of development and function:

I. Primary integration ["social integration"]

II. Unilevel disintegration ["the horizontal dilemma"]

III. Multilevel disintegration: Spontaneous ["vertical crises spontaneously arise"]

IV. Multilevel disintegration: Directed ["the higher is sought, the lower inhibited"]

V. Secondary integration ["autonomous integration"]

THE ROLE OF TRAUMA IN HUMAN LIFE AND DEVELOPMENT

Suffering and trauma are ubiquitous parts of human experience, often leading to intense experiences of grief, anxiety, depression, or feelings of hopelessness (as mentioned, Dąbrowski called these psychoneuroses). Traditionally, psychiatry and psychology have perceived such feelings as symptoms that need to be treated, with the goal of restoring an individual to stability as quickly as possible. Dąbrowski, to the contrary, suggested that crises are *necessary* for growth.

Prior to Dąbrowski, the philosopher Friedrich Nietzsche famously wrote "what doesn't kill me makes me stronger." Others had also begun to see opportunity in crisis. Victor Frankl said that suffering offered an opportunity to develop a feeling of deeper meaning in life. Psychiatrists Eric Lindemann and Gerald Caplan also suggested that one potential outcome of individual crises was personal transformation and growth. Dąbrowski took this thinking one step further and was the first to suggest that crises are actually an essential element in personal development; without crises there can be no growth.

DIFFERENCES IN THE OUTCOMES OF TRAUMA

Dąbrowski concluded that the different outcomes of trauma are determined by the personality characteristics and developmental potential of the individual.

The common pathway to recovery

The socialized individual in primary integration will experience trauma and respond according to social roles and expectations. For example, after the loss of a loved one, various rituals will come into play to help the individual grieve and get over the loss. The average individual generally does not experience any long-term impact from trauma. In the usual course of events, after a brief period of crisis, the individual returns to his or her former level of function—this is psychological resilience. In terms of the antisocial individual, it is said that he or she does not suffer from trauma; rather, such an individual inflicts trauma on others.

Post-traumatic stress disorder

The emergence of the construct of post-traumatic stress disorder has advanced the understanding of long-term negative outcomes from traumatic events. Post-traumatic stress disorder is now recognized as a fairly common outcome of trauma (on the order of 20 percent). Dąbrowski was aware of the possibility of this kind of negative outcome when he described negative disintegration. He saw that some individuals have a constellation of negative personality features—negative developmental potential—that may predispose them to develop long-term adverse impacts from trauma.

Post-traumatic growth

The latest understanding of trauma outcomes has emphasized another possibility: post-traumatic growth. This term was coined in 1995 by Richard Tedeschi and Lawrence Calhoun. As mentioned, after encountering trauma many people display resilience and return to their previous level of function. For others, hardship not only challenges one's character, it brings about a new awareness and appreciation of life. This culminates in personal growth. Dąbrowski essentially referred to post-traumatic growth as positive disintegration.

Dąbrowski was one of the first to advocate for the possibility that trauma could have a positive outcome. Furthermore, he observed that the development of an autonomous personality invariably involved an individual's positive response to intense crises or trauma.

POSITIVE PSYCHOLOGY:
A NEW HOME FOR DĄBROWSKI?

The foundations of positive psychology begin with William James's interest in the subjective experience of the individual. In 1954, Abraham Maslow coined the term positive psychology when he encouraged the study of the virtues, potentialities and aspirations of individuals. Contemporary positive psychology is associated with Martin Seligman and Mihaly Csikszentmihalyi, authors of a seminal article published in 2000. Since then, many psychologists have begun to look at the processes leading to individual development, thriving and flourishing.

Dąbrowski highlighted the important role played by *positive* psychology in his thinking. He said the absence of symptoms was not sufficient to define mental health. Mental health must be defined based on *positive* criteria, and for Dąbrowski, the fundamental cornerstone of mental health is the development of a unique, self-chosen, self-directed, and autonomous personality. This exemplifies the tenets of positive psychology. Combined with the recent construct of post-traumatic growth, Dąbrowski's work yields a powerful approach to personality development.

CONCLUSION

Dąbrowski's theory is based upon a solid foundation of philosophy, psychology, neurology and psychiatry. The theory is challenging because it presents new constructs, including several that seem contradictory until seen in the overall context of the work. This book, *Positive Disintegration*, originally published in 1964, represents an early introduction to the theory. Its continued relevance will be immediately apparent to anyone familiar with contemporary positive psychology and post-traumatic growth. I have no doubt that Dąbrowski would welcome a new audience who would critically review his ideas, update them, and ultimately advance and refine his constructs to better understand and facilitate advanced personality development. To that end, this republication of *Positive Disintegration* represents a timely and essential contribution to the ongoing discussion regarding the transformation of the individual and society.

William Tillier, M.Sc.
Calgary, Alberta
March 2016

Selected Bibliography

Caplan, G. (1961). *An Approach To Community Mental Health.* London, England: Tavistock.

Caplan, G. (1964). *Principles Of Preventive Psychiatry.* New York, NY: Basic Books.

Frankl, V. E. (1985). *Man's Search For Meaning.* (Revised and Updated). New York, NY: Washington Square (Pocket Books). (Original work published 1959)

Harrison, M. K. (1965). Lindemann's crisis theory and Dąbrowski's Positive Disintegration Theory – A comparative analysis. *Perspectives In Psychiatric Care*, 3(7), 8–13. http://doi. org/10.1111/j.1744-6163.1965.tb01446.x

Maslow, A. H. (1954). *Motivation And Personality.* New York, NY: Harper.

Mendaglio, S. (Ed.). (2008). *Dąbrowski's Theory of Positive Disintegration.* Scottsdale, AZ: Great Potential.

Nietzsche, F. (2005). *The Anti-Christ, Ecce Homo, Twilight of the Idols, and other writings.* (A. Ridley, Ed., J. Norman, Trans.). New York, NY: Cambridge University Press.

Seligman, M. E. P., & Csikszentmihalyi, M. (2000). *Positive Psychology: An Introduction. American Psychologist*, 55, 5–14. http://doi.org/10.1037/0003-066X.55.1.5

Tedeschi, R. G., & Calhoun, L. G. (1995). *Trauma And Transformation: Growing In The Aftermath Of Suffering.* Thousand Oaks, CA: Sage.

Tillier, M.Sc., W. D. (2016). *The Theory of Positive Disintegration* by Kazimierz Dąbrowski. Retrieved from http://positivedisintegration.com/

1.

The Theory of Positive Disintegration

The ontogenetic development of man is characterized by factors which appear, increase, reach their peak, and then become weaker and even disappear. This growth and decay, development and destruction, increase and decrease, occurs with emotional factors as well as with intellectual ones, with physiological and with anatomical elements.

Human behavior, from birth through development, maturation, and old age, is under the influence of basic impulses. During the process of growth a particular impulse may weaken, some specific functions of the mind may diminish, the importance of one personal goal might decrease and another assume dominance. Even during the reign of a specific factor, a contrary element may appear which first seems to be a minor side path but slowly becomes the general avenue of development. These diverse tendencies all derive from the biological life cycle.

Throughout the course of life of those who mature to a rich and creative personality there is a transformation of the primitive instincts and impulses with which they entered life. The instinct of self-preservation is changed. Its direct expression disintegrates, and it is sublimated into the behavior of a human being with moral values. The sexual instinct is sublimated into lasting and exclusive emotional ties. The instinct of aggression continues in the area of conflicts of moral, social, and intellectual values, changing them and sublimating itself.

These tendencies and their realization result in deflection and dispersion of the fundamental impulsive forces. The process occurs under the influence of an evolutionary movement which we call the developmental instinct. Stimulated by this instinct the personality progresses to a higher level of development—the cultural human being—but only through disintegration of narrow biological aims. Such disintegration demonstrates that the forces of the developmental instinct are stronger than the forces of primitive impulses. The developmental instinct acts against the automatic, limited, and primitive expressions of the life cycle.

The action which weakens the primitive sets disrupts the unity of personality structure. Thus personality develops through the loosening of its cohesiveness—an indispensable condition of human existence. The developmental instinct, therefore, by destroying the existing structure of personality allows the possibility of reconstruction at a higher level.

In this procedure we find three phenomena which are to some extent compulsory:

1. The endeavor to break off the existing, more or less uniform structure which the individual sees as tiring, stereotyped, and repetitious, and which he begins to feel is restricting the possibility of his full growth and development.
2. The disruption of the existing structure of personality, a disintegration of the previous internal unity. This is a preparatory period for a new, perhaps as yet fairly strange and poorly grounded value.
3. Clear grounding of the new value, with an appropriate change in the structure of personality and a recovery of lost unity—that is, the unification of the personality on a new and different level than the previously existing one.

Transgressing the normal life cycle are new tendencies, goals, and values so attractive that the individual does not perceive any sense of his present existence. He must leave his present level and reach a new, higher one. On the other hand—as described above—he must preserve his unity; that is, he must continue his psychological life, self-awareness, and identity. Thus the development of the personality occurs through a disruption of the existing, initially integrated structure, a period of disintegration, and finally a renewed, or secondary, integration.

Disintegration of the primitive structures destroys the psychic unity of the individual. As he loses the cohesion which is necessary for feeling a sense of meaning and purpose in life, he is motivated to develop himself. The developmental instinct, then, following disintegration of the existing structure of personality, contributes to reconstruction at a higher level.

PRIMITIVE INTEGRATION

Primitive integration is characterized by a compact and automatic structure of impulses to which the intelligence is a completely subordinated instrument. The adaptation to reality in individuals with primitive psychic integration is limited to direct and immediate satisfaction of strong primitive needs. Such individuals either do not possess a psychic internal environment or possess it in only its embryonic phase. Therefore, they are not capable of having internal conflicts, although they often have conflicts with their external environment. They are unaware of any qualities of life beyond those necessary for immediate gratification of their primitive impulses, and they act solely on behalf of their impulses. In terms of Hughlings Jackson's hierarchy of levels, they are at an automatic, well-organized, unself-conscious level of evolution. Inhibition occurs only in a limited way. Under severe environmental pressure these individuals show slight forms of disintegration but only temporarily, for when the stress ceases they return to their former primitive posture of adaptation. They are not able to understand the meaning of time; they cannot postpone immediate gratification, and they cannot follow long-range plans but are limited to the reality of immediate, passing feelings. They are capable neither of evaluating and selecting or rejecting environmental influences nor of changing their typological attitude. Individuals with some degree of primitive integration comprise the majority of society. In psychopathology we find that psychopaths present very primitive integrated structure.

Nevertheless, the compactness of primitive integration has many variations in degrees of stability and in mutability. In normal persons, primitive structure can be changed with some effectiveness by certain conditions. The structure of the individual may contain stronger or weaker dispositions to disintegration and therefore can be influenced by the stresses and strains of life. These environmental factors which affect the disposition to disintegration determine the active, and in some cases accelerated, development of moral, social, intellectual, and aesthetic culture of the individual and of society.

DISINTEGRATION

In contrast to integration, which means a process of unification of oneself, disintegration means the loosening of structures, the dispersion and breaking up of psychic forces. The term *disintegration* is used to refer to a broad range of processes, from emotional disharmony to the complete fragmentation of the personality structure, all of which are usually regarded as negative.

The author, however, has a different point of view: he feels that disintegration is a generally positive developmental process. Its only negative aspect is marginal, a small part of the total phenomenon and hence relatively unimportant in the evolutionary development of personality. The disintegration process, through loosening and even fragmenting the internal psychic environment, through conflicts within the internal environment and with the external environment, is the ground for the birth and development of a higher psychic structure. Disintegration is the basis for developmental thrusts upward, the creation of new evolutionary dynamics, and the movement of the personality to a higher level, all of which are manifestations of secondary integration.

The effect of disintegration on the structure of the personality is influenced by such factors as heredity, social environment, and the stresses of life.

Loosening of structure occurs particularly during the period of puberty and in states of nervousness, such as emotional, psychomotor, sensory, imaginative, and intellectual overexcitability.

The necessity of partial submission of one impulse to the rule of another, the conflicts of everyday life, the processes of inhibition, the pauses in life's activities—all take a gradually increasing part in the transformation of the primitive structure of impulses to a higher development.

Disintegration may be classified as unilevel, multilevel, or pathological; and it may be described as partial or global, permanent or temporary, and positive or negative.

Unilevel disintegration occurs during developmental crises such as puberty or menopause, in periods of difficulty in handling some stressful external event, or under psychological and psychopathological conditions such as nervousness and psychoneurosis. Unilevel disintegration consists of processes on a single structural and emotional level; there is a prevalence of automatic dynamisms with only slight self-consciousness and self-control. The process of decomposition prevails over the process of restoration. In this kind of disintegration, there are no clear and conscious transformational dynamics in the structure of the disposing and directing centers.[1] Prolongation of unilevel disintegration often leads to reintegration on a lower level, to suicidal tendencies, or to psychosis. Unilevel disintegration is often an initial, feebly differentiated borderline state of multilevel disintegration.

The essence of the process of unilevel disintegration may be shown in the following extract from a diary written by a young male patient who presents signs of increased affective and ideational excitability in a period of emotionally retarded puberty:

> I cannot understand what has recently happened to me. I have periods of strength and weakness. Sometimes, I think I am able to handle everything and at others a feeling of complete helplessness. It seems to me at some hours or days that I am intelligent, gifted and subtle. But then, I see myself as a fool.
>
> Yesterday, I felt very hostile toward my father and mother, toward my whole family. Their movements and

---

[1] The disposing and directing center is a set of dynamics determining the course of the individual. It can be at lower, primitive levels of development or at higher levels of moral and social evolution.

gestures, even the tones of their voices struck me as unpleasant. But today, away from them, I feel they are the only people I know intimately.

I often have sensations of actual fear when watching tragic plays and movies; yet, at the same time, I weep for joy or sorrow at what I see and hear, especially when the heroes mostly lose in their struggles or die.

I often have thoughts full of misgivings, anxiety, and fear. I feel that I am persecuted, that I am fated. I have a trick of repeating phrases, like a magic formula, which drives out these obsessive thoughts. At other times, I merely laugh at such notions; everything seems simple and easy.

I idealize women, my girl friends, mostly. I have feelings of exclusiveness and fidelity toward them, but at other times I feel dominated by primitive impulses.

I hate being directed by others, but often I feel no force within me capable of directing my actions.

We see here considerable instability of structure and attitudes, lack of a clear hierarchy of values, lack of signs indicating the "third factor"[2] and the disposing and directing center in action.

In multilevel disintegration there is a complication of the unilevel process by the involvement of additional hierarchical levels. There is loosening and fragmentation of the internal environment, as in unilevel disintegration, but here it occurs at both higher and lower strata. These levels are in conflict with one another; their valence is determined by the disposing and directing center, which moves the individual in the direction of his personality ideal. The actions of multilevel disintegration are largely conscious, independent, and influential in determining personality structure. They are based, in their development, on the psychic structure of the individual and on the arousal of shame, discontent, and a feeling of guilt in relation to the personality ideal. In multilevel disintegration the mechanism of sublimation makes its appearance; this is the beginning of secondary integration.

Multilevel disintegration is illustrated in the following extracts

---

[2] The "third factor" along with the factors of heredity and environment, determines the maturation of a man. It arises in the development of the self, selecting and confirming or disconfirming certain dynamics of the internal environment and certain influences of the external environment. Its presence is evidence of a high level of personality development.

from the diary of a young student training to become a teacher:

> For several years, I have observed in myself obsessions with thinking, experiencing and acting. These obsessions involve my better and worse, higher and lower character. My ideals, my future vocation, my faith to my friends and family seem to be high. Everything that leads me to a better understanding of myself and my environment also seems high, although I am aware of an increased susceptibility for other people's concerns which cause me to neglect or abandon "my own business." I see the lower aspects of my character constantly in my everyday experiences: in decreased alertness to my own thoughts and actions, a selfish preference for my own affairs to the exclusion of other people's, in states of self-satisfaction and complacency . . . a desire to just "take it easy."
>
> Also, I see my lower nature expressed in a wish for stereotyped attitudes, particularly in regards to my present and future duties. Whenever I become worse, I try to limit all my duties to the purely formal and to shut myself away from responsibilities in relation to what goes on about me. This pattern of behavior makes me dejected. I am ashamed of myself; I scold myself. But I am most deeply worried by the fact that all these experiences do not seem to bring about any sufficient consolidation of my higher attitudes, do not influence my "self" to become my "only self." I remain at once both higher and lower. I often fear that I lack sufficient force to change permanently to a real, higher man.

The process of pathological disintegration (adevelopmental) is characterized by stabilization or further involution with a clear lack of creativity, feeble development and retarded realization of goals, a lack of tendency to transformation of structure, and the prevalence of a narrow, partial disintegration process.

Partial disintegration involves only one aspect of the psychic structure, that is, a narrow part of the personality. Global disintegration occurs in major life experiences which are shocking; it disturbs the entire psychic structure of an individual and changes the personality. Permanent disintegration is found in severe, chronic diseases, somatic as well as psychic, and in major physical disabilities such as deafness and paraplegia, whereas temporary disintegration occurs in passing periods of mental and somatic disequilibrium.

Disintegration is described as positive when it enriches life, enlarges the horizon, and brings forth creativity; it is negative when it either has no developmental effects or causes involution.

DISINTEGRATION OCCURRING IN
SEVERAL FIELDS OF MENTAL LIFE

Having described the fundamental kinds of disintegration, we now turn to a short description of the processes of disintegration and the changes they cause in various areas of human life.

Let us begin with the impulses. The most general dynamic, and the ground for others, is the instinct of life and its evolutionary aspect—the developmental instinct. Two groups of impulses are differentiated in ontogenetic development: autotonic and syntonic. Autotonic instincts are egocentric, such as the drive for self-preservation, possessions, and power; syntonic instincts are heterocentric, such as impulses of sympathy, sexual drives, cognitional and religious drives, and social needs. Some instincts appear to be on the borderline between autotonic and syntonic. For instance, the desire for sexual release in its primitive form is an egocentric, autotonic instinct. However, in the course of development it becomes associated with social, syntonic drives. Both autotonic and syntonic instincts are part of the multidimensional instinct of development. The existence of these two opposite groups of instincts, each superimposing itself on each progressive development of the other, provides opportunity for conflicts between them. Every battle between them gives rise to a new balance, a new complex of compromise, a new development of personality.

The effect of positive disintegration on the developmental instinct is as follows: During the embryonic period the developmental instinct is biologically determined. After birth it contributes to adaptation (instinct of adaptation) to the sensing of inner forces in relation to the environment, and to the drive to establish balance between these inner needs and outer realities.

In the next phase of the developmental instinct the instinct of creativity appears. Creativity expresses non-adaptation within the internal milieu and a transgression of the usual standards of adaptation to the external environment. Von Monakow's mechanism of *klisis* and *ekklisis* in relation to the external world (attraction to and avoidance of external objects) is also present in the internal environment. In creativity, there is both a fascination with and a rejection of internal conflicts.

In the further progress of the instinct of development, the personality structure is influenced; this is the phase during which the instincts of self-development and self-improvement emerge. With this phase the "third factor" begins to dominate within the internal environment. There is an extension of creative dynamics over the whole mental structure. Processes of multilevel disintegration (*klisis* and *ekklisis* in relation to certain factors of the internal environment, feelings of shame, guilt, and sin, and an "object-subject" relationship to oneself) appear in the development of personality. We also see an increase in concern with the past and the future and a clear development of a personality ideal.

In this phase of self-development, in which the personality structure is moving ever closer to its ideals, there are two distinct constituents: The first is a dynamic of confirmation, the approval of aims and the ideal of personality; the second is a dynamic of disconfirmation, the strong disapproval of certain elements within the self, and the destruction of these elements. This occurs as the third factor becomes stronger in its effect on personality.

The most obvious aspects of positive disintegration occur in the sphere of feeling. Throughout the thalamic center of the protopathic affectivity, throughout the cerebral centers of emotional life based on an ever stronger stressing of the factors of pleasure and pain, we come upon activities of the highest level, which, shattering the primitive level of affectivity, mix and revalue the fragments, not only building a stratiform division but also releasing new managing dynamics and subordinating previously existing forms. Under the influence of positive disintegration, will and intelligence are separated from each other and become independent of basic impulses. This process causes the will to become more "free" and the intelligence to change from a blind instrument in the service of impulses to a major force helping the individual to seize life deeply, wholly, and objectively. In the further development of personality, intelligence and will are again unified in structure, but at a higher level.

In religious individuals, development produces such signs of disintegration as asceticism, meditation, contemplation, and religious syntony (the feeling of unification with the world). All these are signs of stratified development of the internal environment.

In relating disintegration to the field of disorder and mental disease, the author feels that the functional mental disorders are in many cases positive phenomena. That is, they contribute to personality, to social, and, very often to biological development. The present prevalent view that all mental disturbances are psychopathological is based on too exclusive a concern of many psychiatrists with psychopathological phenomena and an automatic transfer of this to all patients with whom they have contact. The symptoms of anxiety, nervousness, and psychoneurosis, as well as many cases of psychosis, are often an expression of the developmental continuity. They are processes of positive disintegration and creative nonadaptation.

This view indicates that the present classification of mental symptoms and many of the generalizations about them are not satisfactory for the complex, multivarious problems of mental health. The classification and generalizations may suffice for the psychiatrist who deals only with patients coming to him in the psychiatric clinic, but they are inadequate to the handling of problems of prevention, difficulties in child development, problems of education, and minor problems of nervousness and slight neurosis. The "pathological" disorders of impulses, of rationality, and of personality can be, on the one hand, the symptoms of serious illness, noxious for an individual and for society, but on the other hand they may well be—in the author's opinion—and usually are a movement toward positive development. In fact, these disturbances are necessary for the evolutionary progress of the individual to a higher level of integration. Increased psychomotor, sensual, imaginative, and intellectual excitability are evidence of positive growth. These states are frequently found in individuals at times of their greatest psychological development, in highly creative persons and those of high moral, social, and intellectual caliber.

The theory of positive disintegration places a new orientation on the interpretation of nervousness, anxiety, neurosis, hysteria, psychasthenia, depression, mania, paranoia, and schizophrenia.

Let us now turn to the expression of positive disintegration as it occurs in some mental disorders. Hysterics do not have a harmonious emotional life, but very often they have deep emotional relationships to other people and a sensitivity to the feelings both of others and of themselves. They often show a tendency to idealize and present individualistic patterns of intellectual and imaginative activity. They are frequently highly creative. Because of a propensity to suggestion and autosuggestion, they have a very changeable attitude toward reality. Their inclination toward dissociation is unilevel in nature. They do not adapt easily to new conditions. They are moody and display a tendency to overexcitability and depression. Their opinions, work, relationships with other people, and life attitudes are likely to be quite changeable. Besides these characteristics, they have rather infantile psychic traits. The expression of the instincts of self-preservation and sex is, for example, rather superficial and capricious. The lack of multilevel forms of disintegration means the lack of sufficient self-consciousness and self-control.

The psychasthenic, as the name implies, is characterized by weakness. Either physical or psychological asthenia may predominate. Patients in whom psychic asthenia is dominant usually seek help in hospitals and sanatoria; those in whom somatic asthenia is dominant generally try to handle their difficulties themselves. Many in the latter category are writers, actors, and philosophers, often persons performing difficult mental work. In the structure of psychasthenics we often note weakness of lower dynamics with strong higher, creative ones. For this reason the lower level of function of reality (practicality) may be troubled, while the higher level of the same function may be very efficient (creativity).

In both states of cyclic disorders one can observe symptoms which are positive for personality development. The depressive syndrome with inhibition which makes action difficult and gives rise to anxiety and suicidal thoughts is a disintegration of the internal environment. In this phenomenon we see cortical inhibition, an excess of self-analysis and self-criticism, and feelings of sin and inferiority. The manic state shows intensified general feeling, rapidity of thought, emotional and psychomotor excitement, and great mobility of attention. Symptoms of the manic state will vary depending on the hierarchical level attained by the individual. At lower cultural levels there will be aggressiveness, provocation of annoyance, and a tendency to respond to annoyance; individuals at higher levels will show excessive alterocentrism, social hyperactivity, and creativeness. In manic-depressive psychosis the nature of the disintegration will depend on the changeability from manic stage to depression and on the level of culture.

Paranoia is characterized by psychomotor excitability, rapidity of thinking, a great inclination to criticize others without self-criticism, and an intensified self-attention without feelings of self-consciousness and self-doubt. Paranoiacs present a very rigid integration with systematized delusions of persecution and grandeur, and egocentric excitability. They also reveal an inability to adapt to real situations that contributes to a narrow form of unilevel disintegration. The absence of self-doubt and self-criticism and the narrow range of the symptomatology reflect the absence of multilevel disintegration. Paranoid structure to some extent is similar to psychopathic structure in that both show integration. In the psychopath, the integration is broad but is at a low hierarchical level, whereas the paranoiac the integration is at a higher hierarchical level but is partial and thus contributes to narrow unilevel disintegration.

The schizophrenic shows two basic symptoms: intensified mental excitability and psychic immaturity which hinders adjustment to the environment (especially to an unsuitable environment). In schizophrenia there is fragility and vulnerability to external stimuli, psychic infantilism, and weakness of drives. The schizophrenic individual is characterized by hyperesthesia with an inclination to disintegration and very often to accelerated development. Disintegration in schizophrenia is a mixture of positive and negative types on the borderline of multilevel and unilevel disintegration. There are hierarchical traits in levels of integration, but the integration is fragile and has distortions. Schizophrenics are inhibited and rigid and have strong anxiety and autism. The irregularity of environmental influences and the shortening instead of prolongation of the developmental period (perhaps because of a special constitution) lead to intolerance of developmental tension, to negation, and to fragmentation of the personality. Nevertheless, some plasticity of psychic structure and dynamics is present, since it is not uncommon for the psychiatrist, after a long period of observation, to change his diagnosis from schizophrenia to reactive psychosis with some schizophrenic characteristics.

From the point of view of the theory of positive disintegration, we can make a diagnosis of mental disease only on the basis of a multidimensional diagnosis of the nature of the disintegration. The diagnosis may eventually be validated by observation of the eventual outcome. The distinction between mental health and mental illness rests on the presence or absence of the capacity for positive psychological development. Somatic diseases such as cancer, tuberculosis, and heart disease cause psychic disturbances in individuals who are well adapted to both external and internal environments. They permeate a broad or narrow, short or long interval in life activities, an interruption of integrated relations of the individual. The interruption of life activities means that the dominant disposing and directing center is unable to engage in all of its previous activities. This curtailment may lead to a large partial disintegration and withdrawal of one field to another level. The transfer from one level to another is possible only in cases which exhibit a hierarchical internal milieu.

POSITIVE AND NEGATIVE DISINTEGRATION

The positive effect of some forms of disintegration is shown by the fact that children (who have greater plasticity than adults) present many more symptoms of disintegration: animism, magical thinking, difficulty in concentrating attention, overexcitability, and capricious moods.

During periods of developmental crisis (such as the age of opposition and especially puberty) there are many more symptoms of disintegration than at other times of life. These are also the occasions of greatest growth and development. The close correlation between personality development and the process of positive disintegration is clear.

Symptoms of positive disintegration are also found in people undergoing severe external stress. They may show signs of disquietude, increased reflection and meditation, self-discontentment, anxiety, and sometimes a weakening of the instinct of self-preservation. These are indications both of distress and of growth. Crises are periods of increased insight into oneself, creativity, and personality development.

Individuals of advanced personality development whose lives are characterized by rich intellectual and emotional activity and a high level of creativity often show symptoms of positive disintegration. Emotional and psychomotor hyperexcitability and many psychoneuroses are positively correlated with great mental resources, personality development, and creativity.

How can positive disintegration be differentiated from negative disintegration? The prevalence of symptoms of multilevel disintegration over unilevel ones indicates that the disintegration is positive. The presence of consciousness, self-consciousness, and self-control also reveals that the disintegration process is positive. The predominance of the global forms, the seizing of the whole individuality through the disintegration process, over the narrow, partial disintegration would prove, with other features, its positiveness. Other elements of positive disintegration are the plasticity of the capacity for mental transformation, the presence of creative tendencies, and the absence or weakness of automatic and stereotyped elements.

With regard to sequences: The presence of unilevel symptoms at the beginning of the process of disintegration does not indicate negative disintegration to the degree that it would later in the process. The presence of retrospective and prospective attitudes and their relative equilibrium, and the process of the formation of a personality ideal and its importance to the behavior of the individual—these indicate a positive operation.

The capacity for syntony with other individuals (in the sense of emotional closeness, understanding, and cooperation even with the possibility of organized and conscious conflicts with them) also indicates a positive process. In cases of psychoneurosis and sometimes psychosis, in addition to the factors listed above, positive disintegration can be recognized by the individual's capacity for autopsychotherapy.

The criteria of differentiation between positive and negative disintegration must be further studied from the point of view of the diagnostic complex, the characterologic pattern, and the environmental circumstances in which they occur. The points above are only a brief, initial effort at clarifying this problem.

The accuracy of the differentiation of a positive from a negative disintegration process in a specific individual can be proved by examination of the eventual outcome of the process. In the great total process of evolutionary developmental transformation through disintegration, negative processes are relatively infrequent and represent a minor involutional discard.

SECONDARY INTEGRATION

Secondary integration is a new organization of compact structures and activities arising out of a period of greater or lesser fragmentation of the previous psychic structure. Partial secondary integrations occur throughout life as the result of positive resolutions of minor conflicts. The embryonic organization of secondary integration manifests itself during the entire process of disintegration and takes part in it, preparing the way for the formation of higher structures integrated at a higher level. The seeds for integration are the feeling of dissatisfaction, discouragement, protest, and lack of higher values and needs for them. This state increases the sensitivity of the individual to both the external and the internal environment, causes a change in the primitive impulse structure, forces the transformation of primitive impulse structures, and encourages the movement of psychic dynamics to a richer, higher level. As secondary integration increases, internal psychic tension decreases, as does movement upward or downward of the disposing and directing center, with the conservation, nevertheless, of ability to react flexibly to danger. The disintegration process, as it takes place positively, transforms itself into an ordered sequence accompanied by an increasing degree of consciousness. Secondary integration can proceed in different ways: It can be (1) a return to the earlier integration in more nearly perfect form; (2) a new form of integration, but with the same primitive structure without a higher hierarchy of aims; or (3) a new structural form with a new hierarchy of aims. This last form represents a development of the personality.

POSITIVE DISINTEGRATION AND THE DEVELOPMENT OF PERSONALITY

The most important elements of disintegration which indicate future integration and development of the personality are as follows:

1. Definite seeds of secondary integration.
2. Prevalence of multilevel rather than unilevel disintegration, with an attitude of rejection toward "lower" structures.
3. A definite instinct of development with approval of higher structure and dynamics.
4. Strong development of a personality ideal.

Symptoms of disintegration occur in highly talented people. There is a difference between the disintegration process in the development of personality in a subject of normal intelligence and that process in the course of life of a genius. In the normal subject disintegration occurs chiefly through the dynamism of the instinct of self-improvement, but in the genius it takes place through the instinct of creativity. The first concerns the total psychic structure, the second only certain parts of psychic organization.

IMPLICATIONS OF THE THEORY OF POSITIVE DISINTEGRATION

In psychology, this theory emphasizes the importance of

developmental crises and gives an understanding of the developmental role of, for example, feelings of guilt, of shame, of inferiority or superiority, of the "object-subject" process, of the "third factor," and of so-called psychopathological symptoms. It introduces new elements to the present view of the classification and development of instincts. It does not regard instincts as rigid and as existing only under the influences of phylogenetic changes but rather conceives of them as changing through positive disintegration, losing their primitive strength and evolving to new levels of expression in the cycle of human life.

In education, the theory emphasizes the importance of developmental crises and of symptoms of positive disintegration. It provides a new view of conduct difficulties, school phobias, dyslexia, and nervousness in children. An awareness of the effect of multilevel disintegration on the inner psychic milieu is of basic importance for educators.

In psychiatry, this theory leads to an increased respect for the patient, emphasis on psychic strengths as well as on psychopathological processes, and attention to the creative and developmental potential of the patient. The theory indicates the necessity in diagnosis and treatment to distinguish disintegration as either positive or negative in nature. The theory of positive disintegration represents a change in the traditional psychiatric concepts of health, illness, and normality. Perhaps these concepts can be clarified by the presentation and discussion of two case histories.

TWO CASE HISTORIES

Case One

PROBLEM. Ella, 7½ years old, was admitted directly to second grade in a public school on the basis of her admission examination. During the first days of school she had many difficulties. She was emotionally overexcitable, had trouble eating and sleeping, and cried at night. There was a weight loss of five pounds, and she showed some signs of anxiety and transient depression. She asked her parents to transfer her to first grade of the school.

The patient was the older of two children. Her sister, 5 years and 10 months old, was more of an extrovert and more independent than the patient. The mother was harmonious, rather introverted, and systematic in her work. She was concerned about the long-range implications of the patient's difficulties. The father was of mixed type with some cyclic and schizothymic[3] traits. He was dynamic, self-conscious, and self-controlled. The development of both children had presented no special problems. During the preschool period Ella had been an obedient girl but from time to time emotionally overexcitable, ambitious, independent in her activities, and sensitive toward the external environment, though in a subtle, private way. She had always had a great deal of inhibition. At 4½ she had begun to discuss with her parents the problems of loss, of death, and of life after death.

MEDICAL AND PSYCHOLOGICAL EXAMINATION. Medical and psychological examinations were both negative. I.Q. was 128. Rorschach: ambiequal type with some predominance of kinesthetic perceptions. Aptitude toward mathematics, decorative arts, and, in general, manual dexterity was evident. There was a tendency to introversion and systematization of work. The first steps in her work and in a new situation were the most difficult for her. Once they had been taken, she did much better. She was very clearly inhibited, although ambitious, and had feelings of inferiority and superiority.

INTERPRETATION. Ella was an introvert with rather schizothymic traits. She was intelligent, self-conscious, and inclined to be emotionally overexcitable, and her excitability was easily transferable to the vegetative nervous system. She was ambitious and tended to be a perfectionist but was somewhat timid and likely to resign in the face of external difficulties. She had symptoms of transient depression, anxiety, and inhibition. However, her aims and ideals were clear, and she leaned toward moral and social

---

[3] *Schizothymic* is Kretschmer's term. It refers to an asthenic bodily type having such psychic characteristics as theoretical rather than practical abilities, difficulty in contact with people, and some tendency to internal conflict.

concerns. She presented the type of emotional tension very closely related to psychic development.

We see in this case a fairly early stage of positive disintegration with emotional overexcitability, ambivalences, and the initial formation of psychic internal environment. There is the gradual construction of the disposing and directing center, hindered by the child's inhibition but supported by her determination to handle new situations despite anxiety, her strong feeling of obligation, and her ambitions. This conflict, increased by her need to meet a new situation, presents a crisis in development.

TREATMENT. This child must be treated with an awareness of the positive function of her symptoms. In our evaluation we see her as an intelligent and ambitious child with many assets who at present is in a developmental crisis. The wisest course would be to help her surmount this crisis. Her successful handling of the school situation will decrease her inhibition, strengthen her disposing and directing center, and contribute to her further development.

Ella can, and preferably should, be treated at a distance and not through direct psychotherapy. Originally, her teacher had intended to transfer the patient to the first grade. The child knew of this decision, and it had increased her ambivalence; she was depressed and she herself asked to be transferred. However, after a conversation with the psychiatrist, the teacher changed her mind. Understanding the situation better, she helped the child by not asking her to participate in class but allowing her to come forward whenever she felt prepared to answer. In six months she was one of the best pupils in the class and received an award for her work. Emotional tension diminished and the dystonia of the vegetative nervous system disappeared.

There are further means of help. One could see the child from time to time at long intervals, following her normal lines of development and her normal internal and external conflicts. We must know the conditions of her family and school life and perhaps help her parents to be aware of her developmental needs and, on the basis of this understanding, of the ways in which they can help her to more permanent adaptation both to herself and to social life.

DISCUSSION. We have viewed this case as that of a normal child with a high potential for development and have seen this development through a necessary crisis precipitated by a new, difficult external situation. We have not recommended any psychiatric treatment. What might be the effect if these symptoms were seen as psychopathological and treated by intensive psychotherapy? The emotional, introverted, and self-conscious child could be deeply injured. The labeling of the symptoms as pathological in itself would have a negative effect. In addition, the social milieu would be likely to view the child as disturbed if she were seen in intensive psychotherapy, as, indeed, would the child herself. The apprehensions of the parents might increase, and the teacher might treat the child in a more artificial manner than she would otherwise. All this would increase the emotional tension of the child, especially her tendency to an introverted attitude and timidity. These conditions could create new problems and an increasing need for psychotherapy.

Directing Ella's attention to the products of her fantasies could result in excessive attention to them and artificially increase their effect (although knowledge of them would give increased understanding to the therapist). Regarding the symptoms as psychopathological would imply the desirability of their elimination. However, they perform a positive function for this child, and to deprive her of them would be a serious matter. Focusing on pathology might accentuate anxiety, inhibition, and flight into sickness. Viewing and treating these symptoms as psychopathological would itself create conditions that would appear to confirm the correctness of that approach.

Case Two

PROBLEM. Jan, a 21-year-old student of the Polytechnic Institute, came to the Mental Hygiene Clinic with his problem: He had failed twice to pass from the first to the second year of classes. He had symptoms of depression and thoughts of suicide. The patient was very close to his mother and in states of depression would announce that he would commit suicide if his mother died. He was afflicted with speech disturbance—stuttering. He felt unable to complete examinations with groups of students since he was anxious about his stuttering and concerned that he would be ridiculed. Under these circumstances, he found himself unable to concentrate on his examinations.

MEDICAL AND PSYCHOLOGICAL EXAMINATION. Neurological, laboratory, x-ray, EEG procedures were all negative. The patient was extremely intelligent and particularly apt in his field of studies. He showed a high emotionality and imaginative overexcitability, strong inhibitions, guilt, an attitude of timidity, discontentment with himself, feelings of inferiority toward himself, and feelings of disquietude and anxiety. He presented a very strong moral structure and a tendency to be exclusive in his emotional attitude and in his relation to other people.

Jan's father had died when he was 10 years old. He had one brother eight years older than himself. Jan's past history showed the gradual development of his symptoms. During puberty at 15 years of age, they were particularly strong but in time receded. It was during this time that he first showed a slight stutter. This minor speech defect had tended to decrease since then, but it had lately abruptly increased.

Further information revealed that he was in love with a high-school girl of 17, but he was sure that she did not love him. However, he had no objective basis for this conclusion. His timidity had prevented him from declaring his interest. The mother, who had heart disease, was sympathetic to her son and wanted him to be married. The relationship with his mother was particularly strong because he did not have other confidants.

Jan's depression had begun to deepen when he felt he had failed in his love affair and especially after his second failure in his examinations. There was an increase of inferiority feelings toward himself and of feelings of distance from and meaninglessness of the external world.

INTERPRETATION. The patient was introverted, schizothymic, and emotionally overexcitable and had trouble adapting himself to the demands of the external environment. He was very inhibited and had an inferiority complex based on his stuttering. He had a high level of subtlety of introspection and moral attitude toward himself and his environment. There was a clear hierarchical development of the psychic internal environment, but his disposing and directing center was not strongly developed because of lack of attainment of his aims, poor adaptation to this social environment, and lack of proper self-evaluation. In the various difficulties of everyday life his emotional excitability increased, and he showed the symptoms of subacute emotional crisis. This state caused, and was in turn increased by, his difficulty in taking examinations and his subsequent failure. At the same time, his condition was clearly connected with his emotional attachment to a girl and his inability to realize a satisfactory relationship with her.

Psychoanalytic therapy might be very helpful to this patient, although a narrow psychoanalytic approach might focus too exclusively on his relationship with his mother and particularly on his hostility and guilt. Of course, this young man had guilt with regard to his mother and we could discuss here his Oedipus complex. But this was not the core of his difficulty; it was, rather, related to the development of his personality. In the development of personality the psychic internal milieu grows through the dynamism of multilevel disintegration. Guilt is one of many useful dynamisms, as are discontentment with oneself, feeling of inferiority, and disquietude. Jan's examination of himself in relation to his mother, his concern about his fantasies, and his feelings of special obligation because of his mother's illness all contributed to a sense of distance between his lofty ideals and obligation and his feelings of the inadequacy of his everyday life. This guilt can lead to a greater self-knowledge and clear ideals. No man develops a high level of personality without this process.

TREATMENT. After a conversation with the psychiatrist, the Dean of the Faculty allowed the patient to be examined alone, rather than with a group. A social worker saw the girl in whom he was interested. It was clear that she knew of his interest and loved him, but, being of the same type of timid and inhibited personality, she had difficulty in expressing her feelings.

Jan was given speech therapy and psychotherapy. The

psychotherapy was aimed at helping him understand and utilize his character pattern and symptoms. In his type this meant the recognition of and collaboration with the principal dynamics of his development. Thus it was necessary to recognize and clarify his introversions, withdrawal from people, vulnerability, and emotional overexcitability. These must be taken up in the context of actual, current situations. Psychotherapy here must encourage a deeply optimistic attitude toward symptoms. This does not mean that the psychiatrist suggests to the patient that he be foolishly cheerful; he must instead develop insight into his inner conflicts and external difficulties and a broad perspective on his future course through the harsh and often indifferent demands of life.

Under the conditions of the new examination Jan passed to the second year, and in the next examination he was one of the highest students in the class. In the course of psychotherapy a new disposing and directing center developed, owing to a decrease of his inhibition, heightened awareness of his own ability, and increased confidence from what he had learned in examining his developmental history. After several years he married the girl with whom he was in love. The marriage led to a new period of life, new problems, and further development.

The treatment did not resolve all of Jan's basic problems, but it helped him to handle the acute crisis and to avoid some tendency to negative disintegration.

DISCUSSION. We see in this patient, an intelligent man, the process of multilevel positive disintegration, which on the one hand makes him capable of accelerated development but on the other leaves him susceptible to developing crises. His psychic distress was on the verge of being psychopathological; it had the potential for either positive or negative disintegration. It indicated deep dissatisfaction with his internal and external milieu and a tendency with very high emotional tension to resolve this on a higher level of synthesis. His symptoms could be diagnosed as "mixed depression and anxiety neurosis" or perhaps "borderline schizophrenia," but such a label is merely psychiatric etiquette.

Since we see in Jan the progressive development of himself through external and internal difficulties, this patient is regarded as mentally healthy. From the point of view of the theory of positive disintegration, psychotherapy is multidimensional aid in overcoming too severe a crisis in the positive development of man.

2.

The Principal Dynamics
of Multilevel Disintegration

In the preceding chapter, the theory of positive disintegration was described, and multilevel disintegration was distinguished from unilevel. But such a survey automatically denies detailed consideration of the manifold dynamics of multilevel disintegration itself: the feeling of disquietude, shame, discontentment with oneself, guilt, inferiority feelings toward oneself, and "subject-object" attitude.

DISQUIETUDE

The disquietude arising from the attitude of the individual toward his own development is completely different from the disquietude which arises in the same individual from concern about his security within the environment. The second stems from the primitive instinct of survival, the first from the development of the internal psychic environment. The individual feels responsible for his own development; his sensitivity in regard to this feeling of responsibility (originating from concern that the growth of his personality is insufficient) results in a restlessness about himself. This disquietude presents an element of great importance for personality development and is very close to the process of astonishment in the evolution of intellectual activities. Disquietude and the astonishment of discovery are creative dynamics in the primary phase of development: the first is involved with the growth of feeling, the second with intelligence. Disquietude is a sign to the individual that his mental activities are in some way defective in reaction to external stimuli and are thus inappropriate. This new awareness is a signal of the birth of a direction center at a superior level; it is the symptom of the loosening and disorganization of the internal psychic environment. It reflects a discordance of primitive impulses integrated at a low level and of the tendencies which are not stabilized but voluntary and which have a potential for development. The feeling of disquietude is the first phase of distinction between "inferior" primitive impulses and dynamics of the personality ideal.

SHAME

The feeling of shame is a strong emotion. It arises in a psychic structure sensitive to the reaction of the external world, particularly to environmental disapproval of one's behavior. The presence of this feeling shows that the individual is conscious of the reaction of other people, especially those close to him. It is characterized by excessive response to the moral opinion of others. The sentiment of shame is concerned with internal moral attitudes and with social "opinion" toward these attitudes. In manifesting shame the individual is, to some extent, showing awareness of his inappropriate character. The substance of this feeling is clearly different from that of the feeling of guilt and the feeling of sin. Shame is the primary expression of sensitiveness to the judgment of the external world. It expresses disquietude concerning possible disharmony between moral values of the individual and the values of others around him. It marks one of the first stages of loosening and disintegration of primitive structure and instinct in the process of multilevel disintegration.

The feeling of shame is often expressed by the vegetative nervous system in a predominance of sympathetic reactions, such as acceleration of the pulse and blushing. From the psychic point of view, a shyness, awkwardness and a tendency to retreat are evidenced.

DISCONTENT WITH ONESELF

The feeling of discontent with oneself is the expression of an increase in multilevel disintegration. In the new, broader field of psychic multilevel structure one group of elements becomes the object of discontent and another group the source—one the judged, the other the judge. The first is disapproved by the disposing and directing center; the second is approved. The disapproval is repeated very often with participation of emotional experience of "subject-object" in the psychic internal milieu. Discontent with oneself is the symptom of lack of approval of the activities of primitive impulses. It is an evidence of the birth and development of what is "self" and what is "not self" in the internal environment. Discontent participates in the movement of the disposing and directing center to a higher level of development and in the increase in action of the third factor.

GUILT

The feeling of guilt is the expression of a stronger engagement of the individual with regard to his own conduct than is the case in discontent with oneself. Guilt involves discontent with oneself and in some feeble degree a feeling of shame; it permeates the whole personality and is closely related to affective memory and a retrospective attitude. However, the conscious awareness of his having behaved wrongly, either toward one's own development or toward the human environment, is primary.

Guilt is often expressed by self-accusation and relieved through punishment and expiation. It is a powerful, penetrating feeling, close to Kierkegaard's "fear and trembling," and is connected with compelling movement at both conscious and unconscious levels. Its roots can be found in heredity and in distress in the early ages of life. Guilt has a tendency to transform itself into a feeling of responsibility, which embraces the immediate environment and even all society. As has been mentioned, it seeks punishment and expiation. These latter factors play a major role in relieving the feeling and in beginning the ascent of the individual to higher levels of development.

The sense of guilt arises during the process of multilevel disintegration because it is the expression of a dissatisfaction of the disposing and directing center with some lower activities in the psychic internal environment. Everyday experience and clinical observation have shown that psychoanalytic theories concerning the origin and development of guilt are not justified in many cases. This feeling appears in and is often closely related to strong emotional structure showing great sensitivity in moral and social areas. That is, the individual who has very distinct capabilities of positive development and responsibility is likely to suffer feelings of guilt. This kind of emotional structure is much stronger in nervous and in neurotic individuals. Intelligent and emotionally overexcitable children with a high level of reflection and self-observation often show external and internal conflicts accompanied by the feeling of guilt. For example:

> P—, a 3-year-old girl, very intelligent (I.Q. = 140), impulsive, imaginative, and emotionally hyperexcitable, had a clear attitude of opposition to but at the same time a deep affection for both her parents. Although there was strong mutual confidence between her and her parents, she presented mood changes with egocentrism to which her parents were in opposition. She reacted to the position of the parents by crying. However, a change occurred in this development. Without any coercion from her parents, but on her own initiative, she began to muffle her cries by placing her hands over her mouth. She declared she did not want to be a "crybaby" (the word utilized by the parents at the times of her crises). She rejected this baby crying and said she would be a very "good girl." Her father said at one time that it sounded as if her cries were going up the chimney. After this, whenever she had a tendency to cry, she opened the chimney flue and waited for her crying spell to go away.

SUBJECT-OBJECT PROCESS

In the conduct of the child described in the preceding section we can observe the subject-object process—a normal aspect of positive disintegration in which two structures are opposed to each other in self-differentiation. In this case, one structure was connected with the "good girl," the other with the "crybaby." The child used "magic" to eliminate the unwanted structure. She also showed the feeling of guilt and of responsibility in viewing her "other" self as wicked.

> The same girl, at the age of 6, went to her father and asked him to reach a robe that was on a high shelf, out of her reach. She said that her mother had agreed she could have it. The father was not sure the mother had actually consented, but he accepted the child's statement and gave the robe to her. When the mother came into the room, the lie was discovered, and the girl broke into tears. She did not want to eat and became very nervous. The mother suggested to the girl that she go to her father and ask his forgiveness. The father was very willing to forgive; he said that he very much loved his little daughter but he was surprised that she did not always tell the truth. In asking her father for forgiveness, the child offered all her chocolates to her parents. She assured them she would not take any of these chocolates as she had on other occasions even when she had said that she would not. Later the same evening, her father asked her if she had had a cup of tea. She answered, "Yes." But after a few minutes she began to cry and said, "Papa, I have lied for the second time."

This is a child with psychic overexcitability, of mixed type (emotional, imaginative, psychomotor, and mental) with cyclic and schizothymic traits. Inclination to perseveration, and sensitivity to the stimuli of the external world and to moral and psychological problems are evident.

Discontent with oneself, shame, and guilt, as well as the attitude of retrospection and prospection, are illustrated here. The discontent arises from disharmony between very impulsive activities and attitudes of reflection, which in turn stem from self-consciousness. Self-consciousness and the feeling of guilt lead to differentiation of superior from inferior levels of the internal milieu. The sense of guilt is an indispensable factor in development and particularly springs forth in individuals during rapid development. It contributes to the creative tension which forms the basis of self-education.

Feelings of inferiority and the third force play primary roles in the formation of the psychic internal environment and in multilevel disintegration. These dynamics are helpful both in organizing and in moving the disposing and directing center to a higher level. They participate both in the development of personality and in the clarification of the personality ideal. Since they demand detailed clarification, they will be taken up in the following two chapters.

The operations of "subject-object" become clear when all introspective activities of the individual are taken into consideration. This ability to evaluate various aspects of the self can be understood by examination of its differential activities connected with the internal experiences of the individual. In multilevel disintegration this dynamic of "subject-object" plays a part not only in the internal development of tension but, even more important, in the multiple changes in time and space which result in hierarchical movement and in the elaboration of a new disposing and directing center as it gradually reaches new and higher levels of development. "Subject-object" is closely related to the processes previously discussed: disquietude, shame, discontentment with oneself, feelings of guilt, and inferiority feelings toward oneself. These processes are, to some extent, the expression of object-subject forces in the psychic internal environment. Such forces increase the intensity of all processes acting in the internal psychic environment.

As discussed above, disintegration causes the movement of the disposing and directing center to either higher or lower levels but with a gradual tendency for stabilization at a superior level of development. To the degree that the disposing and directing center takes its place at higher levels, the individual begins to live more closely in accordance with his own personality ideal. The personality, during its formation, not only recognizes its ideal more clearly but takes part both in the elaboration of this ideal and in its effect on the transformation of inferior structures. Localization of the disposing and directing center closer to the personality ideal often occurs in a state of concentration and meditation, particularly after either very difficult periods of life—tragedies and severe stress—or significant pleasant events. Intuitive elaboration of the substance of experiences develops as a result of this transformation.

3.

The Feeling of Inferiority Toward Oneself

TWO CONCEPTS OF INFERIORITY

The feeling of inferiority toward oneself is not discussed in scientific and popular literature. Inferiority feelings which are discussed in the literature are those related to the environment— for example, feelings of worthlessness as compared to others. The problem of inferiority feelings toward the environment, its causes, development, sublimation, and social compensation have been well described by Alfred Adler.

The concept of inferiority toward oneself involves an understanding of the structure and dynamics of the internal environment. The development of this feeling depends on the development of awareness in the internal psychic milieu of values, that is, the ability to distinguish some actions as "superior" and others as "inferior." The sense of values provides a standard of measure for behavior and gives inner support or disapproval to one's own actions.

For the formation of a feeling of inferiority toward oneself another dynamic is necessary: the "object-subject" relationship to oneself, an important factor in the construction of a multilevel internal environment. From this concept we come to the fundamental idea of the process of multilevel disintegration. In the course of positive disintegration we see disquietude in relationship to oneself, feelings of shame and guilt, feelings of inferiority toward oneself, and object-subject relationship to oneself. In this group of dynamics one of the most important is the feeling of inferiority toward oneself.

According to Adler, the child, having a very feeble and labile psychic structure, has feelings of inferiority in relation to adults, who appear to him to be omnipotent. His sense of inferiority tends to be compensated for by the development of a will to be strong or by excessive submission or aggression. The presence of some handicap, such as an injured leg or ugliness, increases the possibility of the formation and development of the sentiment of inferiority toward the external environment. Inequality and injustice, humiliation, the fact of being an orphan, poor living conditions—all contribute to the growth of this sentiment. The unique or spoiled child may also develop feelings of inferiority toward his environment when he moves from a setting well adapted to him to a different one which fails to recognize his uniqueness, as, for example, when he begins school.

Adler states that feelings of inferiority can be compensated for in social or asocial ways, both of which are often observed. In individuals inclined to self-criticism and with a strong instinct of development, we see the formulation of high goals and observe the phenomenon of a positive, social compensation. There is wide agreement with the opinion of C. M. Campbell: "There are not many accomplishments of humanity that do not involve the feeling of inferiority."[4] Intellectual development and the development of moral and social personality are impossible without the participation of this form of inferiority feelings, but feelings of inferiority toward oneself are also involved.

Positive disintegration occurs in every global development of man, especially during periods of accelerated development. It is a process of loosening and often of temporary dissolution of psychic structure, as in psychoneurosis and, more rarely, in psychoses. Multilevel disintegration is closely related to psychoneuroses and nervousness. It is also related to increasing self-awareness through the perception and elaboration of pleasant and unpleasant experiences.

---

[4] *Towards Mental Health: The Schizophrenic Problem.* Cambridge, Mass.: Harvard University Press, 1933.

The feeling of inferiority toward oneself is one expression of the process of multilevel disintegration, and it arises from the greater self-awareness and the self-examination that occur in multilevel disintegration.

The fundamental differences between feelings of inferiority toward the external environment and feelings of inferiority toward oneself are in the words *toward the external environment* and *toward oneself.* Feelings of inferiority toward the external environment present a phenomenon which can be permanent or temporary in all human beings—those who are normal, neurotics, psychopaths, and persons having many different psychotic disorders.

The feeling of inferiority toward oneself generally appears in individuals capable of development, especially accelerated development. It is manifested in nervousness, in psychoneurosis, and in psychosis, but it does not appear in psychopaths or in paranoid individuals.

The sentiment of inferiority as regards the external environment is related to conflict with this environment. The sentiment of inferiority toward oneself, when it is not morbid, constitutes a prophylactic factor in relation to the external environment. It is expressed and is a symptom of moral and cultural development. In contrast, the feeling of inferiority toward the external environment is primitive and occurs earlier in psychic development. It is not connected with development of the internal environment, whereas inferiority feelings toward oneself are very strongly bound with the existence and the increasing development of the internal milieu.

HIERARCHICAL LEVELS

Awareness of the structure and dynamics of the internal environment is generally closely related to disintegration, especially to multilevel disintegration. In normal people this consciousness usually develops during the periods of puberty and menopause. It appears when internal conflicts are present, under conditions of suffering, and in psychoneuroses. The internal environment is intimately coupled with the development of a hierarchy of feelings, that is, an awareness of different levels within oneself. The experience of hierarchy is much clearer during periods of change in one's values, either ascending or descending from previous levels.

Emotional knowledge of the internal milieu is associated with awareness of this hierarchy and with the movement of the disposing and directing center. This emotional experience contributes to the development of a consciousness which distinguishes many levels of values and many qualities of structure within the internal milieu. The feeling of inferiority toward oneself is connected with awareness of "infidelity" toward the personality ideal. It arises in the descent from a high level of values to a lower one.

The feeling of hierarchy—the awareness of multiple stratification—in oneself cannot occur without a clear personality ideal and a realization of the distance of many aspects of this ideal in the areas of impulsive, emotional, and intellectual activities. The very awareness of one's hierarchical levels is often the source of the feeling of inferiority toward oneself in the course of development. This occurs in periods of decrease in moral activities and in the comparison of the present level with the previous higher levels of behavior. The individual who is developing at a high level cannot always be without a moral disruption within himself and some degree of negative progress.

Individuals are not always at the highest level of their development. Fatigue, nervousness, disquietude, and anxiety may cause them to descend to lower levels of activity, that is, to a more primitive integrated state. But the individual in real development cannot remain at this level long. He becomes discontented with himself; he has feelings of guilt and of inferiority toward his personality ideal. He then has the tendency to return to his higher level of development. The "fear and trembling" described by Kierkegaard is accompanied by conviction of descent from one's proper level.

ROLE OF THE THIRD FACTOR

As more intensive development of the personality occurs, and the disposing and directing center rises to a superior level, the third factor begins to play a greater role in development than does heredity or social environment. As we know, the third factor is an instrumental dynamism of man. Besides taking a negative or affirmative position with regard to one's own behavior, this factor takes a fundamental part in all periods of transformation in which new values replace old ones in the process of the complication and evolution of conscious life. The actions of choice, of negation and affirmation, with regard to the internal and external environment are very closely connected to the feeling of inferiority. In emotional experience, a negative attitude is regarded as inferior and an affirmative attitude is felt to be superior. The third factor constantly participates in all experiences of comparison of the personality ideal with the structure of the disposing and directing center, and with the direction and level of conduct in everyday life. The feeling of distance of this ideal from present activities determines the activity of the third factor and its support or disapproval of present pursuits.

SELF-EDUCATION

Without the feeling of inferiority toward oneself no process of self-education is possible. For self-education there must be a conscious personality ideal and a desire to ascend to this ideal. It is accomplished through increasing organization of the disposing and directing center, which activates the third agent and its obsession for evaluation of present levels of feelings and activities. Exploratory behavior in either "lower" or "higher" directions, with increasing conscious awareness, guides the individual to clearer resentment of inferiority feelings and toward transformation of himself through self-education. Awareness of those things he has and has not realized is often the basis of the creative tension that moves him toward a stronger process of self-education. Self-education leads to the emotional experience of dualism in oneself, that is, an attitude of "object-subject." The attitude expresses the relationship between what is educated and what educates.

The differentiation of inferiority feelings as sick or healthy depends on their place in the total structure and dynamics of the individual and especially on whether they play a creative or noncreative role in the development of the personality. Feelings of inferiority have a positive role in the process of disintegration when disintegration participates in the creative formation of the personality, in the realization of the personality ideal, in the movement of the disposing and directing center to a higher level, and in the increase in activities of the third factor. This is positive utilization of inferiority feelings. The nonpathological feeling of inferiority is generally associated with transformation of the internal psychic environment. It is associated, too, with a creative attitude of negation and affirmation toward specific values of the internal milieu and toward certain forces of the external environment. The feeling of inferiority in the internal environment of the creative individual and the sentiment of inferiority in connection with the social environment, without simultaneous attitudes of resentment and hate toward this environment, express a favorable prognosis for the energy of the individual to be directed to positive transformation. The feeling of inferiority toward the external environment is negative, or pathological, when it has much more strength than the feeling of inferiority toward oneself. In this situation, which occurs in psychopathy and in some psychoses, there is direct expression of aggressive tendencies.

INFERIORITY AND CREATIVITY

The majority of very creative, eminent individuals in the moral, artistic, and scientific areas of life show in their dynamics the development of the sentiment of inferiority toward themselves. Michelangelo, Dostoevsky, St. Augustine, Gandhi, and many others had feelings of inferiority as a basic mechanism. In Proust, Kafka, Żeromski, and other creative psychasthenics inferiority feelings are a fundamental dynamic. Beers and Fergusson, who represented the American movement in the reform of psychiatry and mental hygiene, passed through mental illness and suffered from ambivalent feelings of inferiority and superiority.

Without feelings of inferiority and positive disintegration the possibility of effective realization of the personality ideal and the achievement of a higher level of personality development does not exist. Self-education does not occur without the presence of inferiority feelings in relation to both the internal and the external environment—especially the former. A state of creative psychic tension does not exist without resentment of the distance between the personality ideal and the actual conduct of everyday life. This distance is clearly related to the feeling of inferiority in the internal psychic milieu, particularly with reference to the personality ideal.

4.

The "Third Factor" in the
Development of Personality

Along with inborn properties and the influence of environment, it is the "third factor" that determines the direction, degree, and distance of man's development. This dynamic evaluates and approves or disapproves of tendencies of the interior environment and of the influences of the external environment. It cooperates with the inner disposing and directing center in the formation of higher levels of individuality. Because of the third factor the individual becomes aware of what is essential and lasting and what is inferior, temporary, and accidental both in his own structure and conduct and in his exterior environment. He endeavors to cooperate with those forces on which the third factor places a high value and to eliminate those tendencies and concrete acts which the third factor devalues.

CONCEPTUALIZATION OF THE THIRD FACTOR

The importance of self-objectivity, self-criticism, self-control, and objective evaluation of the social environment has long been recognized. The conceptualization of this force as the third factor not only emphasizes its importance but allows us to more clearly trace its growth and development. This basic element in determining a man's development has a place next to that of heredity and environment. Moreover, its significance increases in the higher stages of man's development. The appearance and growth of the third agent is to some degree dependent on inherited abilities and on environmental experiences, but as it develops it achieves an independence from these factors and through conscious differentiation and self-definition takes its own position in determining the course of development of personality.

The following illustration of the third factor is based on the autobiography of a patient, W—, a student of philosophy, suffering from symptoms of anxiety psychoneurosis:

> I have chosen my "self" from among many "selfs," and I find that I still must constantly make this choice. For many years, during everyday activities, I have found myself questioning which is my "true self," the one I think of as true or another which seems more and more strange to me?
>
> In spite of these self-examinations, my "strange self" appears very strong and may be the cause for my fear of it and my concern for what is the truth of my internal make-up. But I persist in choosing my "true self." Often I am able to discover that certain types of activities belong to my "true self" and others do not.
>
> My immediate environment is of little help to me because (except for a few people spiritually close to me) my environment itself is generally strained. I have a tendency to be opinionated, yet manifest uncertain attitudes in moral problems. These habits tend to provoke hostility about me.
>
> However, when my anxieties weaken and my "true self" gets stronger, it is easier for me to endure pressure from my "strange self" and the effects of my external environment. I become stronger and, at the same time, more serene.

EMERGENCE OF THE THIRD FACTOR

The third agent manifests itself in its initial phase during childhood. We may observe in a child's conduct simple and direct symptoms of his discontent with himself and his behavior; we note that the child seeks forgiveness for incurring displeasure. Manifestations of a child's independence of his surroundings and a growing excitability of a mixed type, with imaginative, psychomotor, emotional, and sensorial components, testify to the germination of the third agent. That is, symptoms of childish nervousness (which are forms of disintegration) express to some extent the activities of the third agent. All that influences the beginning of an accepting and rejecting attitude toward stimuli of the internal and external environment, and the placing of a high value on one inner trait and a negative value on another may be considered embryonic forms of the third agent.

The principal periods during which the third agent appears distinctly are the ages of puberty and maturation. The attitude of affirmation and denial, just beginning to bud in childhood, becomes dynamic at the age of puberty. An increased emotional, psychomotor, imaginative, sensorial, and intellectual excitability favors the process. A young man experiencing a certain loosening of his internal and external environments observes both these environments more or less closely and manifests an attitude of "subject-object" toward his own self. He assumes a critical attitude toward himself and his surroundings, strives to verify opinions with reality, attempts to transmit personal moral experiences to others, and makes demands of a moral nature both on himself and on other people. The consciousness of his ambivalences arouses in him alternately a sense of superiority and of inferiority, a feeling of guilt and self-discontent, and a more or less strong anticipation of the future or retrospection over past experiences. During the period of puberty, young people become aware of the sense of life and discover a need to develop personal goals and to find the tools for realizing them. The emergence of these problems and the philosophizing on them, with the participation of an intense emotional component, are characteristic features of a strong instinct of development and of the individual's rise to a higher evolutionary level. In the period of puberty, therefore, the third agent is more dynamic and conscious than it was in childhood but remains still relatively uncertain in its service to the poorly outlined and wavering disposing and directing center.

The age of puberty moves slowly into a stage of mental harmony, during which time a more stable interior equilibrium arises as well as a greater harmony with the environment. Gradually a new structure forms, integrated on a different and more mature level than the preceding one. The desire to gain a position, to become distinguished, to possess property, and to establish a family will become the disposing and directing center. But the more the integration of the mental structure grows, the more the influence of the third agent weakens. The third agent may even pass away altogether.

The third agent persists—indeed, it only develops—in individuals who manifest an increased mental excitability and have at least mild forms of psychoneuroses. In these persons the disintegration process is protracted, moral ideals continue to play a considerable role, and the inner directing and disposing center continues to be wavering and uncertain, ascending and descending. They display mental liability, excessive naiveté, freshness of feeling, and what might be called the enduring of certain infantile features of the prolongation of the period of puberty. Mental disequilibrium, a certain inclination to normal disintegration, the absence of the swift attainment of a stabilized psychic structure, and a strong third factor are all signs of the ability to develop one's personality toward the realization of one's ideal.

The persisting and growing force of the third agent in adults appears simultaneously with the protraction of the period of maturation, with all of its positive and some of its negative qualities. This extension of the maturation period is clearly accompanied by a strong instinct of development, great creative capacities, a tendency to reach for perfection, and the appearance and development of self-consciousness, self-affirmation, and self-education.

PERSONALITY AND POSITIVE DISINTEGRATION

Personality is a self-conscious, self-affirmed, and self-educated unity of basic and positive mental properties. It is a unity capable of gradual quantitative changes of particular properties and of groups of properties. Qualitative changes may also occur in the personality's process of development, but they are generally marginal as concerns their localization and disposition in relation to basic, already self-conscious and self-affirmed qualities. The formation of personality depends upon the existence of positive processes of disintegration in a given individual, upon the level of the disposing and directing center, and upon the personality ideal.

As we know, positive disintegration may be unilevel or multilevel. The former appears independently or precedes the latter and is then its primitive phase, denoting a loosening of the individual's mental structure with only slight participation of his consciousness. Multilevel, positive disintegration is a conscious process of differentiation of the individual's internal environment and will lead successively through conflicts between "lower" and "higher" levels of the inner environment, through a loosening and sensitization of various dynamics of this milieu, through the mechanisms of feelings of self-discontent, inferiority, and guilt, and through slighter and partial disorders of mental balance to secondary integration—that is, to a mental structure on a higher level.

Secondary integration accompanies dramatic experiences connected with the oscillation of the inner disposing and directing center. The center may descend to a lower level and return (after some time) to the preceding one or it may pass the latter and settle permanently on a higher level.

The third factor appears embryonically in unilevel disintegration, but its principal domain is multilevel disintegration. Disintegration activities are related to the activities of the third agent, which judges, approves and disapproves, makes a choice, and confirms certain exterior and interior values. It is, therefore, an integral and basic part of multilevel disintegration. It is a sort of active conscience of the budding individual, determining what represents a greater or smaller value in self-education, what is "higher" or "lower," what does or does not agree with the personality ideal, and what should be the course of internal development.

THE PERSONALITY IDEAL

Secondary integration is preceded by the formation of a personality ideal, which actively influences the movement of the disposing and directing center to a higher level. The personality ideal is a remote pattern of which the individual is aware. At the same time, it is a store of organized and active forces arising out of multilevel disintegration and secondary integration. The evaluation of the presence and nature of the personality ideal is ascertained by the intuition and simple judgment of every individual realizing self-education; we may, however, conceive of it only in general outline and as a whole.

The disposing and directing center of a developing personality is a more or less organized mental structure, emerging from as yet indistinct tendencies to attain a higher cultural and moral level. These tendencies are directed toward a level higher than the one existing under the immediate influence of environment and of moral standards. With the strengthening of the disposing and directing center, instincts achieve a higher level of expression and consciousness becomes richer. The third agent takes part in the activity of consciousness which determines general motives and evaluates activities as proper or improper. This aspect of consciousness has strong emotional components that participate in the mental and voluntary affirmation or negation of one's general, vital attitudes.

The appearance and development of the third agent parallels the organization and establishment of the disposing and directing center on a higher level and the distinct formation and steady growth of the personality ideal. The third agent draws its dynamics and purpose from the disposing and directing center and the personality ideal; in turn, it plays an essential part in the development of both of them. This is a deeply correlated, reciprocal activity. Generally speaking, however, the position and activity of a higher level of inner disposing and directing center are superior to those of the third agent.

In summary, we may say that the personality ideal provides the dynamic goal toward which the individual directs various mental energies. The disposing and directing center on a higher level constitutes the focus of the structure and dynamics of the arising personality. Disintegration is the mechanism of the process of personality formation. The third factor is subordinate to the personality ideal and to the disposing and directing center on a higher level. It is also a constituent part of multilevel disintegration. The third factor strives to see that every concrete act of a given individual is in correlation with his personality ideal.

The individual human being, through his personality, masters his impulses. This process consists in purifying the primitive animal elements which lie in every impulse or group of impulses. For instance, within the range of the instinct of self-preservation, it will mean the separation and disapproval of lower-level self-preservation tendencies and of what is egocentric—that is, the selfish, indiscriminate striving toward the realization of one's own aims, with no consideration for the good or harm of others. As far as the sexual impulse is concerned, its exclusively somatic, uncontrolled, unindividualized expression, which lacks any tendency to exclusive emotional ties, will be disapproved.

The effect of the third agent is to insure the personality's mastering of its life impulses. It is not limited to acts of choice but takes energy from primitive, sublimated impulses and directs the personality toward creativity and self-perfection.

THE THIRD FACTOR AND THE SOCIAL ENVIRONMENT

During the period of the development of the third agent the individual slowly but essentially alters his attitude toward his social environment. His relation to his environment becomes more and more conscious, clear, and determined. He selects from it elements on which he places value. He becomes more independent. Owing to the activity of the third agent, he begins to accept only those influences of a social group that are congruent with his self-consciousness—those, therefore, that agree with the demands of his developing personality. Hence, in his exterior activity there may occur various forms of nonadaptation and conflicts expressing inner disapproval of those elements in the social group which are not congruent with his personality ideal. Such an individual will often be considered unsocial, queer, unadapted, and difficult. This estimate is incorrect, for the person acting under the influence of the third agent displays basic syntony and cooperation with the needs of social life despite his attitude of contradiction and disapproval.

An alterocentric introversion, or—according to Rorschach— contacting introversion, is usually characteristic of such a person.

SELF-EDUCATION

Self-education is the process of working out the personality in one's inner self. Self-education begins with positive disintegration and the appearance of the third agent. Self-determination then starts to replace heterodetermination little by little. The difficulties of adaptation as well as the development disorders can be removed by means of auto-psychotherapy. From this moment on, moral evaluation and the individual's relation to his environment begins anew, so to speak; the past becomes, in a certain sense, isolated from the present and the future.

In the initial phase of self-education the individual is suspended between the influence of clearly lower impulse tendencies, the strength of which gradually declines, and the pull of the personality ideal and the disposing and directing center, which are only gradually forming and establishing themselves. This is the phase of stratified disintegration, the period of Kierkegaard's "fear and trembling," when one is unable to find support either in the so far primitive impulse dynamics and the "normal" forces of the social environment or in a high level of personality dynamics. This period may be regarded as a time of moral and individual maturation.

The period of real, essential moral maturation is often one of spiritual void: of isolation, loneliness, and misunderstanding. It is the time of the "soul's night," during which the then existing sense of life and forms of connection with life lose their value and force of attraction. The period will close, however, with the working out of an ideal, the arising of a new disposing and directing center, and the appearance of forces of disapproval, shutting out every possibility of a return to the initial level. This is the process of development of personality. The third agent, having now gained the right to be heard, will admit no retreat from the road ascending to a personal and group ideal. The growing realization of a personality ideal is the secondary phase of self-education and is unique to the formed personality.

From the discussion above, we see clearly that the third factor plays a vital role in the development of psychic inner environment. Its action is very closely connected with multilevel disintegration, especially with the development of an "object-subject" process within the self. It participates in the establishment of a disposing and directing center at a higher level and in the development and organization of a hierarchy of psychic structure and of the personality ideal. This structure and these dynamisms are necessary to self-education and autopsychotherapy in internal conflicts and to positive development in psychoneurosis.

5.

Remarks on Typology Based on the Theory of Positive Disintegration

On the basis of the theory of positive disintegration we can distinguish some dynamic character complexes with reference to patterns of developmental transformation. Four character patterns can be identified: primitive integration type, positive disintegration type, chronic disintegration type, and pathological disintegration type.

PRIMITIVE INTEGRATION TYPE

This character pattern is a stabilized, primitive level of integration in which development of personality does not take place. Its occurrence seems strongly influenced by constitutional factors.

In the pattern of primitive integration, frequently seen in everyday life, the disposing and directing center may have strong impulses, the direction of which decide the course and forms of behavior. The individual's relationships with others are impulsive in nature and not influenced by self-awareness. He responds to external stress with only a slight degree of disintegration. The tragedies of everyday life, such as the death of parents or friends, loss of a job, and imprisonment, are likely to produce only mild symptoms of disintegration. The disposing and directing center may fragment slightly but, because of the stable, compact integration, remains at the previous level. The individual returns to his everyday habits and activities; his difficulties will not have contributed to any transformation of his original psychic structure. When change of personality occurs, it is related to disintegration during psychic and physical development. This does not happen in persons of the primitive integration type.

Psychopaths are among those with primitive integration structure. They are characterized by a stable integration at a low level, and their activities clearly reflect primitive impulses. They are insensitive to stimuli other than those related to their psychopathic structure of impulses. This type of individual is not aware of the feelings of other people; syntony never develops. Intellectual activity is clearly of instrumental character and subordinated to lower-level impulses.

Among normal primitively integrated people, different degrees of cohesion of psychic structure can be distinguished. The tendency to develop disintegration may be present in greater or lesser degree, but the elements of disintegration are much more feeble than the forces of integration. However, external stress, a high level of intelligence, and a capacity for introspection can help loosen the psychic structure and thus increase the potential for growth. Another life course may be distinguished in this type, for the forces of disintegration arising out of the experiences of life can result in a partial development. This, however, is rare.

The following is an example of primitive integration:

L—, a male engineer aged 34, was a specialist in a narrow field of technical science. There was nothing distinctive about either his heredity or his early development. His parents were rather simple people, normally ambitious in their outlook for the future of their children. L—showed good progress during his early school years. He was himself ambitious to excel in order to rise to a higher position. He was reasonably accommodating and sociable but showed little interest in the concerns of other people. From his childhood, he had been rather selfish in this way, caring primarily only for his own affairs.

After his secondary schooling and the completion of his technical studies (where again he obtained good grades) he went on to specialize in his field. He progressed very rapidly and soon gained a favorable opinion among his superiors, partly through his abilities and industry, but for the most part because of his principle of avoiding conflict with his colleagues and superiors. He devised several methods of flattery adapted to the varied levels of his environment. These methods were well worked out and effective, but quite primitive.

After several years of experience in his field L— perfected what seemed to him an infallible system of acquiring the protection of higher authority, a system based on four basic principles: first, avoid all conflict with colleagues, thus reducing their sense of competition; second, flatter authority, specifically praising the "creative" ability of a superior; third, help both colleagues and superiors, but within limits so that personal time and effort are never exhausted; and fourth, carefully deprecate, in the presence of superiors, the value of scientists in other fields.

As mentioned above, L—had abilities, but they were incommensurable with the speed of his career. His weaknesses he countered by adjusting the tempo of his work and employing an enterprising "sixth sense" to catch and use any means whatever that might accelerate his career. Certainly it was to his advantage that he had specialized in a narrow field of science, poorly developed in his own country. His immediate superior had ambitions of his own: to initiate and expand this field of science in the country by creating a group of student-disciples.

L—devoted all his time and efforts to obtaining, as soon as possible, a high rank in this narrow field. To this end he conformed all his needs of friendship and love. He deliberately did not marry in order to avoid any obstacle in his career. By the judicious application of his four-part system he soon earned the reputation of cleverness.

L's personal ambitions increasingly restricted his scope of experience and interests. His syntony was superficial, even artificial, subordinated to the main aim of his life. There remained in him a distinct feeling of inferiority to those who, in his opinion, had reached a still higher level in the social hierarchy. On the other hand, he did not reveal any feelings of self-dissatisfaction. He did not feel inferior in regard to any internal ideal. He had no sense of guilt, despite his hypocrisies. In fact, the attitude of striving toward any moral ideal seemed strange to him. His guiding principle of life was to accommodate himself to changing conditions in order to take advantage of them for his personal benefit.

In spite of his amiability and sociability, he was emotionally cold. He had no ability to transfer his own feelings to other people or theirs to him.

His single external conflict was simple envy, the sense of inferiority in the presence of his social superiors. His life until the age of 34 was that of a person integrated on a low impulsive level with his intellect fully subordinated, used as a tool in his drive toward a higher rank—a "career" in the common meaning. He had no internal depth, no distinct germs of moral personality. Rather, he showed signs of disappearing traces of the higher dynamics mentioned above. For that reason, L—was not subject to the process of positive disintegration.

POSITIVE DISINTEGRATION TYPE

This character pattern reveals the process of loosening and fragmentation of psychic structure, and transformation through the displacement of previous values and the introduction of new values. Multilevel disintegration is closely related to the development of the psychic environment. An individual of this type feels anxiety with regard to his own values and deep dissatisfaction with himself. He reacts to feelings of guilt and of inferiority toward himself and shows awareness of "subject-object" relationships to himself.

The positive disintegration type develops progressively through the life cycle by the processes of positive, multilevel disintegration. The individual is highly sensitive to the stimuli of both internal and external psychic environments and has the capacity to comprehend and accept a hierarchy of values. He reveals attitudes of both retrospection and prospection, a depth of experience due to a rich emotional memory. He is consciously aware of personal and social ideals and capable of mobilizing them. Because of past internal progressive transformations, he can understand and collaborate with individuals of various personality patterns. He has the ability to understand many different levels of development in others. Such a person is often involved in conscious and controlled conflict with the external world. All these qualities contribute to a high level of values and an exceptional degree of maturity.

CHRONIC DISINTEGRATION TYPE

In the positive disintegration type can be seen many levels of achievement. The level attained depends on the higher and higher organization of the disposing and directing center, increasing self-consciousness, and progressive mobilization of the energy of the personality ideal on the path to secondary stabilization. Besides the positive disintegration type described above there is a chronic disintegration type, which manifests different characteristics. An individual of this type experiences multilevel disintegration but without definite tendencies to secondary integration. While he does not have the propensity to achieve synthesis of the decomposed structure, he shows no signs of psychopathological deterioration. However, crystallization of the processes of secondary integration is lacking. In the chronic disintegration type there is significant loosening and fragmentation of psychic structure but no noticeable development of an active disposing and directing center. An individual of this type is inclined to perpetual oscillation between different dynamisms and continual changing of activity and positions. He is incapable of decisive and determined behavior. Oscillation is his major characteristic. In the continuous variation of impulses which change his responses to external stimuli, no predominant stabilized value can be observed. This type is creative and reveals some hierarchy of values, but this too varies. Such a person may be, at the same time, productive and inhibited, impressed with moral and social values and skeptical of them. He is without vital direction because of his hesitant attitude; at times he does not see any value in life or in creative activity. He has his own preventive forces against involution: the processes of positive disintegration and creativity. Although he does not develop strong mental disorder, he is seldom able to achieve secondary integration.

PATHOLOGICAL DISINTEGRATION TYPE

In this type of development there is negative disintegration: a decrease of consciousness and an increase of destructive processes with a tendency toward involution of the total personality, as in the chronic organic psychoses and the chronic schizophrenic psychoses. The psychic structure gradually fragments, the sphere of consciousness diminishes, and there is a loss of creative capacities. Of course, in this type of disintegration many subtypes can be distinguished.

Through the dynamics of positive disintegration development can progress from lower to higher types. The contrary can occur through the processes of negative, pathological disintegration. In the primitive integration pattern, there is little possibility of transformation to another type.

The cyclic individual possesses intellectual, moral, and aesthetic potentialities which form a solid basis for personality development. In this type of person positive disintegration will result in the diminution of exaggerated sociability, overly practical attitudes, opportunism, and strong adaptation to the external environment. Positive disintegration in this type also leads to increased independence from the external environment (which little by little builds a hierarchy of values) and a heightened inclination to solitary meditation.

The contrary is true of the schizothymic type: Positive disintegration will lead to the development of some interest in other people, certain adaptations to the external environment, and some diminution of the feeling of exclusiveness of one's own norms. Thus such an individual will develop the capacity for symbiosis with other people.[5]

Transformation and development in the individual with imaginative overexcitability often occur. Indeed, a person of this type has the potential for considerable development. Through positive disintegration he will deepen his imagination and at the same time enlarge his sensitivity to the external world of nature and of social life. He will develop tendencies to evaluate and limit his impetuous, incorrect observations. As he enlarges his sense of reality, he will increase the degree of organization of his psychic structure. This form of transformation will permit him to build a heterogenic psychic structure in which intellectual, psychomotor, emotional, and sensory elements will help to deepen his imagination.

---

[5] The effect of positive disintegration on Jung's extrovert type is similar to its effect on the cyclic type discussed above; and its effect on Jung's introvert type is similar to the discussion of the schizothymic type.

6.

Psychopathy and Psychoneurosis

In terms of the theory of positive disintegration, psychopathy represents a primitive structure of impulses, integrated at a low level. The intelligence is subordinated to this structure and plays the role of an instrument. The psychopath possesses a strong constitutional factor, low sensitivity to other people's attitudes, and strong egocentric dynamics; he is indifferent to everything except his own small needs. The psychopath does not experience the anxiety one sees in the psychoneurotic; he does not suffer conflict in his internal milieu. In other words, he never undergoes a period of multilevel disintegration. Therefore, he neither is conscious of the complexity of his internal environment nor sees himself objectively. He is incapable of either self-criticism or self-control.

Without positive disintegration the psychopath's disposing and directing center remains primitive while it dominates the intelligence. The lack of a disintegration process is the chief reason for the psychopath's lack of syntony. He has no awareness of "we" but only a strongly developed sense of "me." His adaptation to the environment is accomplished by the instrumental acts of his intelligence, not by his capacity for experiencing or his insight into the structure and dynamics of other people. As a result of this primitive structure, a psychopath is an asocial and, under the influence of his primitive directing center, often an antisocial individual.

The psychoneurotic individual differs from the psychopath.

He is sensitive, restless, and capable of somatic expression of mental process through his vegetative nervous system. Often shy, apprehensive, and dissatisfied with himself, he has feelings of inferiority and guilt and may display a feeling of inferiority with regard to his environment. He experiences within himself the "subject-object" process—an increased self-awareness and an introspective knowledge of the many levels of his own personality. This is a process of experiencing one's own being, so to speak, of sensing one's own multiform nature which determines the process of cognition as well as of experiencing. The psychoneurotic's personality is plastic and variable since he is in a dynamic state of awareness of the subtleties of both his internal and his external environment. He is, therefore, a personality capable of disintegration and has the ability for distinct and often rapid development.

The psychoneurotic may have conflicts in relation to his external environment, but usually his conflicts are internal ones. Unlike the psychopath, who inflicts suffering on other people and causes external conflicts, the psychoneurotic himself usually suffers and struggles with conflicts in relation to himself. In contrast to the psychopath, a psychoneurotic has a strong self-consciousness. As stated above, the psychopath's lower (impulsive) mental dynamics are integrated, whereas the psychoneurotic displays a disintegration not only of primitive levels but even of middle and high development levels. The psychopathic individual is able to develop only to a minimal degree; only if he has some neurotic factor in his psychopathic structure is there any possibility for personality development. The psychoneurotic, however, is capable of continuous evolutionary development through the process of disintegration and subsequent secondary integration.

THE DISPOSING AND DIRECTING CENTER

The disposing and directing center in a psychopathic individual is integrated at a low level. This center consists of a dominating impulse or group of impulses directing the individual's life aims. Often intelligent, the psychopath is sometimes able to disguise his aims and patterns of behavior, but they nearly always reveal a low level and primitive quality.

In psychoneurotic persons the disposing and directing center presents quite a different aspect. In view of the disintegration, particularly the multilevel disintegration, characterizing psychoneurotics, the disposing and directing center remains in a more or less unstable position. For a certain period it may be stabilized at a low structural level; later, it may pass on to the middle level. Finally, in periods of stronger development of personal ideals it may localize itself on a higher level. General weakness, emotional fatigue, and loosening of mental tension may sometimes lead to a periodic stagnation, even at a low level of integration, whereas constant insight into one's own interior environment (which is characteristic of the disintegration process), restlessness, self-dissatisfaction, feelings of guilt, sin, and inferiority toward oneself—the sources of increased tension—may bring the psychoneurotic individual to a higher level of integration.

The disposing and directing center has, therefore, no fixed level in psychoneurosis; it is unstable, migrating from one level to another, with a prevailing tendency to settle at a higher level. In states of disintegration (especially unilevel disintegration) over a period of time the psychoneurotic will reveal a multiplicity of directing centers and a change in their level. During puberty, for example, psychic movement can be observed between feelings of superiority and inferiority. A psychoneurotic will demonstrate rapid changes in values, ambitendencies, and ambivalences.

The lack of stability of the disposing and directing center in psychoneurosis and its distinct stabilization at a low level of emotionally cognitive structure in psychopathy are clearly connected with the problems of structure and function of the internal environment. In truth, we can hardly speak about internal environment in psychopathy, since the level of self-consciousness of psychopaths is very low. The psychopath is not subject to the process of multilevel disintegration. All his activities are strictly subordinated to impulsive dynamics at a low level.

THE FEELING OF INFERIORITY

Although the psychopath does not undergo any essential processes and experiences characteristic of multilevel disintegration, he may experience a feeling of inferiority. But it is a feeling of inferiority with regard to the *external* environment, not a self-dissatisfaction. A contrary phenomenon occurs in psychoneurotics. Such individuals demonstrate various types of increased excitability. Psychoneurotics are typical examples both of the process of development of internal environment and of the process of disintegration, especially the multilevel type. All the above-mentioned processes, which are lacking in psychopaths, are characteristic of psychoneurotics.

Essential elements of psychoneurosis are the dynamization of the internal environment, the experiencing of hierarchy in oneself, and the strong manifestation of dynamics progressing toward an ever higher hierarchy of values up to the personality ideal. With a growing awareness and stabilization of his personal ideal, the individual becomes more conscious of the distance separating him from it; his sense of reality increases, and the dynamics leading to the realization of his ideal become more distinct. As the personality develops, the substance and dynamics of the ideal become the principal disposing and directing center in the individual's development—the main source of developmental energy.

THE THIRD AGENT

What is the role of the third agent? The third agent, together with the first agent (inherited and inborn dynamics) and the second (environmental influences), becomes the major developmental agent in highly cultured individuals with a high degree of self-consciousness. The dynamics of the third agent arise and develop in a certain number of individuals during periods of stress and during the developmental crises of life such as puberty, adolescence, and the climacteric. Rudiments of this agent may be seen in especially talented, sensitive, and sometimes nervous children. The third agent functions to deny some and affirm other specific peculiarities and dynamics within the individual's internal environment, at the same time denying and affirming certain forms of influences of the external environment. The third agent selects, separates, and eliminates heterogeneous elements acting in both internal and external environments. The third agent becomes active during periods of strong tension of the developmental instinct and during positive multilevel disintegration. It operates in individuals endowed with strong tendencies toward positive development and, therefore, may be often seen in nervous, neurotic, and psychoneurotic persons. Such individuals often have inferiority feelings (typical of these disorders), connected as a rule with the process of disintegration.

In psychopathy, there is neither a process of disintegration nor the development of a third agent because the disposing and directing center consists of an impulse or group of impulses integrated at a low level. Nor does the psychopath experience inferiority feelings with regard to himself because the development of this feeling presumes the process of disintegration.

INTELLIGENCE

The disposing and directing center guiding all the psychopath's activities consists of primitive impulses to which the intelligence is subordinated as an instrumental adjunct. Moreover, it is a very strong subordination, permitting absolutely no transformation into self-critical activity.

The situation is quite different in psychoneurosis. The disintegration process characteristic of psychoneurotics sets in action multiform, multilevel, changeable conjunctions of intelligence with various disposing and directing centers which repeatedly move toward an ever higher level. In emotional, as well as intellectual, activities processes take place which lead to a purposeful loosening of the different levels of intelligence activity. Hence, in both neuroses and psychoneuroses conjunctions of disposing and directing centers with the activities of intelligence are multiform and variable.

POSSIBILITIES OF DEVELOPMENT

Psychopathy is a rigid structure of largely constitutional character on a low level of integration with no essential ability for positive development. One might admit certain possibilities of development under very strong and early influence, the action of which would cause the loosening or breaking up of the primitive impulsive structure. This influence would have to create some internal conflicts and anxiety within the psychopath, the first step in the development of the internal psychic environment. But such an eventuality is rather unlikely.

Nervousness and psychoneuroses are structures and groups of functions especially likely to develop positively by processes of unilevel and multilevel disintegration. Without these processes no positive development of a human individual is possible. Without nervousness and psychoneuroses there is no positive disintegration, and without positive disintegration there is no development.

CREATIVE ACTIVITIES

Psychopaths as a rule do not create cultural works. The psychopath's intelligence, even at a high level, is not of a creative nature; it merely serves the egotistic purposes of the dominating impulse or group of impulses. Hence, even extensive use of intelligence leads not to creative ideas but to destructive action. As a result of these strong impulsive dynamics, it is difficult for the psychopath to make a long-range, controlling estimate of his own and other people's acts; therefore, he has no capacity for sympathetic insight into the states of mind of others and is unable to grasp any social, moral, or cultural problems.

Psychoneurotics, on the contrary, create works of culture because of their high moral sensitivity, their capacity for introspection, their ability to estimate their own and other people's attitudes, and their ability to differentiate levels and to experience the "subject-object" process within themselves, i.e., because of their susceptibility to the processes of disintegration, especially those of multilevel disintegration.

In connection with these remarks, it is pertinent to quote a passage from Proust's novel *Le Côté de Guermantes*: "All that is great we owe to neurotics. They, and no others, have founded religions, created masterpieces. The world will never know how much we owe them, and especially how much they suffered to give all this to the world. We glory in their divine music, their beautiful paintings, and thousands of subtleties, without realizing the innumerable sleepless nights, tears, spasmodic laughters, urticaria, asthma, and—worst of all—fear of death they cost those who created them."

Professor Neyrac, speaking about the role of fear in the life of Saint-Exupéry, the French author and aviator, said, "This was a fear of a special kind, having the property of raising the personality's development. Such fear is an instrument for raising to a higher level, and physicians should approach it with prudence and respect."[6]

---

[6] Quoted in Abély, P. De quelques équivoques psychiatriques. *Ann. Medicopsychol.* (Paris), 117:46–78, 1959.

7.

Jackson's Theory and Positive Disintegration

Hughlings Jackson, the famous English neurologist, early in his career fully resolved to give up medicine and devote himself to philosophy but later decided to continue his medical career. His interest in philosophy led to his careful analyses of neurological symptoms and to major theoretical contributions that have served for many decades in the interpretation of psychological, psychopathological, and neurobiological phenomena. Jackson's work can be summarized in three principles which describe evolution from three points of view, each harmonizing with the other.

THREE PRINCIPLES OF EVOLUTION

The first of Jackson's hypotheses is that evolution is the transfer from a perfectly organized lower center to a higher but not so well-organized one. In other words, development consists of movement from lower, comparatively well-managed centers to higher centers that are more complex and, according to Jackson, less well organized.

The second principle is that evolution is a transition from the simplest to the most complex, from the lowest to the highest centers. There is no contradiction in regarding the most complex centers as being the least organized, since Jackson uses the word *organized* to mean well-connected. "Let us consider," says Jackson, "a center composed of two sense and two motor elements, the former and the latter so well-connected with each other, that every excitement transfers easily from sense to motor elements. The organization of this very simple center is, nevertheless, on a very high level. We may also imagine a center composed of four sense and four motor elements, but the connections between these elements being so imperfect that it proves to be only half so well-organized as the former one."

The third of Jackson's principles of evolution is that evolution is a transition from a more automatic to a more voluntary center. He assumes that the highest centers, representing the summit of nervous evolution and forming the physical basis of consciousness, are least organized, although most complex and voluntary.

DISSOLUTION

As far as the negative process, or dissolution, is concerned, Jackson writes that dissolution is a process quite the reverse of evolution. It is a process of involution, so to say, contrary to development: Dissolution proceeds from a more complex, voluntary, and not so well-organized center to a simpler, more automatic, and better organized one. Jackson in principle speaks only about partial dissolutions since total dissolution would be equivalent to death.

Partial dissolution may involve a given level or several levels of the nervous system, in a larger or smaller degree, or it may concern only a distinctly limited field. The first kind of dissolution, broader in scope, is generally related to mental disorders, the second to neurological ones; the first belongs to the field of psychiatry, the second to that of neurology. In addition, Jackson distinguishes positive and negative symptoms of dissolution. While negative symptoms appear as a consequence of disturbance of higher levels of the nervous system and signalize loss of function, positive symptoms are the results of activity of lower levels of the nervous system, not affected by disease. These are conceived as compensation for the damaged activities at higher levels of the nervous system.

Mental or nervous diseases are thus manifested directly only by negative symptoms and always begin at the most highly developed level, growing in a succession contrary to evolution. Concerning Jackson's theories, Mazurkiewicz[7] says, "All positive symptoms are not occasioned by disease, but are normal activities in lower levels, set free, owing to a lack of suppression from superior levels."[8]

Dissolution, as above mentioned, may occur at various levels. The first level is characterized, according to Jackson, by lack of equilibrium and by alterations of personal unity manifested either by inner conflicts or by an emancipation of the unconscious system (by which Jackson means the expression of automatic behavior beyond the control of personality, such as tics and some compulsions). A feeling of manifoldness in one's inner self, automatisms, juxtapositions of parts of one's body, a feeling of strangeness toward oneself (kinesthetic states)—these are the expression of a deeper dissolution process. Jackson's commentators consider these states to be a disappearance of differences between subject and object.[9] The patient subject to mania displays a consciousness of unlimited activity, an identification of himself with the wave of time and the universe. Ey and Rouart regard the inability of a patient to adapt to surrounding reality as one of the negative symptoms of numerous morbid disorders.

The basis of Jackson's theory is the principle of the hierarchy of subordination and the dissolution or regression of the structure of functions. Personality, according to Jackson, ought to be considered as the total of an individual's tendencies, beliefs, emotions, and mental activities and capacities. It is the result of biological heredity, of physical structure, and of the psychological drama in which the individual has taken part.

The similarities of some processes occurring in normal people and pathological symptoms has led several authors to the concept

---

[7] Mazurkiewicz, who died in 1946 in Warsaw, was an outstanding Polish psychiatrist in the field of Pavlovian psychiatry and a neo-Jacksonist. His work was in the area of qualitative changes in the development of the nervous system and on the significance of emotions as directing forces in the life and development of both animals and human beings.

[8] J. Mazurkiewicz. An Introduction to Normal Psychophysiology. (Wstep do *Psychofizjologii Normalnej.*) Warszawa: PZWL, 1950. Vol. I, p. 358.

[9] H. Ey et J. Rouart. *Essai d'Application des Principes de Jackson a une Conception Dynamique de la Neuropsychiatrie.* Paris: F. Alcan, 1938.

of normal dissolution. For example, sleep is seen as having several degrees of dissolution: drowsiness, sleep with dreams, active sleep (somnambulism), and sleep without dreams. Ey and Rouart judge that all the three latter forms of sleep are an expression of dissolution in higher brain centers.

ORGANIZATION OF THE HIERARCHICAL SYSTEM

As we know, Jackson's theory is based upon a multilevel analysis of the nervous system. His concept of a well-organized center on a low level of hierarchy is easy to understand; it is more difficult to accept the statement that higher centers are less well organized than lower ones. By the term *good organization* Jackson seems to mean simplicity and automaticity. Yet "good organization" is not to be identified only with simple and automatic functions; it may also take place in a complex, labile structure. The good organization of a given system or a given center consists in the efficient execution of its tasks, and this may characterize a lower as well as a higher center. Here is an example taken from Forel, and quoted by Mazurkiewicz and Frostig: "The author, in order to stop a fight between two tribes of forest ants, dropped a speck of honey in the path of ants hurrying from their ant hill to the fight. The majority of the army of ants did not stop to taste the honey; and those who did stop did so for only a short moment."[10] Although it would seem that the social instinct of combat in ants is a more voluntary, younger structure than the instinct of self-preservation or food gathering, it appears to be at least as well organized as the latter. It is difficult, therefore, to accept Jackson's belief that a less organized center could subordinate a better organized one. In people capable of development, lower, simpler centers are mostly subordinated to a higher, more complex center.

Jackson does not inform us what the essential processes of evolution are and by what activities shifting takes place from a simpler center to a more complex one, from a more organized to a less organized center, and from an automatic to a voluntary center.

---

[10] Mazurkiewicz, op. cit., p. 302.

Mazurkiewicz[11] and other authors consider that development proceeds by superposing new dynamics on top of old ones and not by destruction of the latter; therefore, the evolution of directing dynamics is at the same time a process of their increasing complexity in the directions pointed out by Jackson. Mazurkiewicz clearly stresses the fact that Jackson's theory ought to be extended by accepting qualitative differences between activities of different levels of the nervous system. He states that without this "an evolution from impulse to will" is not conceivable, as every impulse is an action depending until recently on a stimulus whereas voluntary actions always depend on one's own activity— and therefore on past rather than present stimuli. "The forces of the external world and the tendencies of the organism," Mazurkiewicz writes, "expressed by its own activity may not be reduced to a difference of quantity."

> The evolution of activities of the whole nervous system is dynamically an evolution advancing from a mixed, muscular-receptor nervous cell that appears already in coelenterates and the action of which depends only and exclusively on external stimuli, up to the adult human brain which is part of the nervous system, but anatomically distant from the periphery and functionally only very indirectly linked with it. This results, among other things, in the possibility of its displaying intentional management and will in a manner remote from the simple transmission of impulses along the reflex arc.[12]

Those qualitative differences of actions are closely connected with particular areas of the nervous system, in which, according to Jackson, three layers may be distinguished: spinal cord and medulla oblongata, which is most automatic and firmly organized and has only slight voluntary processes: striate body and Rolando's area; and gyri of the frontal cortex. Obviously the number of levels, as well as of qualitatively different mental strata, may be conceived by authors in various ways. It is just these qualitative differences that represent antagonism between the activities of particular levels. Mazurkiewicz describes this process: "in these cases we have to do

---

[11] *Ibid.*, p. 295.
[12] *Ibid.*, p. 258.

with two antagonistic forces of a rather unstable equilibrium, with the prevalence of the evolutionally younger dynamics, but with the possibility of preponderance of the older dynamics under certain conditions."[13]

The example of the ants above quoted proves the transient, unstable equilibrium of antagonistic forces (hesitation observed in a few ants stopping for a moment by the honey drop) and also shows in the majority of these insects an indisputable prevalence of a factor of later development (social instinct) over the more primitive one (alimentary drive). Mazurkiewicz is of the opinion that the development of dynamics is accomplished by their "superposing" over the old ones, not by the destruction of the latter. It is possible that new dynamics destroy the old ones; however, it would seem that the "unstable balance" occurring between the activities of particular levels, i.e., the antagonism described above, may occasion severe alterations in older structures as a result of the growing significance of new ones.

EVOLUTION THROUGH POSITIVE DISINTEGRATION

What are the processes of evolution, and by what steps do we pass from simple reflexes, connected with external stimuli, to complex behavior? In contradiction to the views of Jackson and the neo-Jacksonist school represented by Mazurkiewicz, many mechanisms designated in the theories of Jackson as dissolution play a principal role in evolution. We call them processes of positive disintegration. This raises the question of the role played by disadaptation in the individual's development, including disadaptation to internal as well as external environment. It seems that in the process of evolution the factor of conflict with the surroundings and one's own self has a prominent part in checking primitive impulses. Reflection, hesitation, and inhibition, instead of automatic reaction to stimuli, are the expression of disadaptation; and these generally precede the gradual process of adaptation to new external and internal conditions. Such an unstable equilibrium gives the

---

[13] *Ibid.*, p. 101.

opportunity for the maturing of a new disposing and directing center. Hence, internal and external disadaptation, the absence of direct response of motor elements to stimuli, and the multiplying of indirect links between stimulus and reaction may increase the possibility of new and higher-level functioning and greater creativity. This whole process may result in a gradual development of new centers and new psychic paths—contrary to the opinion of Jackson and the neo-Jacksonists, who regard all mechanisms of dissolution as morbid. On the basis of the analysis of many groups of symptoms, it is evident that such a shifting of forces leads to psychoneurosis, which, in my opinion, is not morbid but rather one of the primary paths to positive evolutionary development. This evolution is not in contradiction to many mechanisms of dissolution but involves them, dissolution forming a basic mechanism of the evolution.

Dissolution can involve those lower, more primitive forms of memory, emotions, and impulses which are not included in the immediate level of the patient's aims. I disagree with the Jackson-Mazurkiewicz position that in mental disease there is always compensation for injured higher activities by a superactivity at lower levels. Mazurkiewicz has said that "memory is a feature of every one of the three basic psychic dynamics (cognition, emotion and psychomotor activity). Each develops during mental evolution, and may, therefore, be simple or more complex, well-or-badly-organized, and similar to a reflex or nearer to conscious and voluntary activity, according to Jackson's law."[14] It must, however, be added that lower kinds of memory may be subject to dissolution, owing to the influence of superior conscious activities.

Psychiatrists, encountering in their scientific and clinical work mental disorders of great intensity which often end unfavorably, have identified general morbid mechanisms in slighter mental disorders—psychoneuroses, states of depression, fear, anxiety, and lack of mental equilibrium—with mechanisms in drastic processes of involution. This is why psychiatrists attach an exaggerated meaning to any symptoms that are similar to those

---

[14] *Ibid.*, p. 128.

appearing in various morbid processes. It seems probable, however, that many of the slighter disorders just mentioned are an expression of positive developmental processes. For what is the path of evolution? It follows partial disintegration, which leads to the formation and conflicts of contrary sets of tendencies, then moves toward the development of a complex, multilevel structure with the formation of a higher hierarchy of aims.

Jackson's error (augmented by Mazurkiewicz) concerning the rejection of qualitative differences between different levels of the nervous system continues to be made whenever the psychiatrist overlooks qualitative differences in the mental disorders of various developmental levels. States of depression and hypomania, delusional symptoms, feelings of strangeness in relation to the world and to the self will differ qualitatively from one another and will have different meanings, depending upon the level of development on which they appear. Jackson, distinguishing negative and positive symptoms of dissolution, did not perceive that among positive symptoms we often encounter those which lead to the development of a higher evolutionary level. This is illustrated by the passing from feelings of inferiority and guilt through a state of disharmony and the conflict between various sets of tendencies to a level of stable moral values.

In his last paper Mazurkiewicz quotes the view of J. Joteyko concerning the participation of conflicts and inner disharmony in the development of man: "Mental states have a life of their own; they strive to live and develop fully. This being their aims, they fight inextricably, the winner triumphing. Those states cannot co-exist without struggling in our consciousness, which always represents one whole, but whose field of vision is limited to one spot. The aim of that fight is to assure the very best functioning of mental activities by perfecting its elements and by the victory of the strongest."[15] These strenuous contests and conflicts, described as "over-educated self-consciousness" by Żeromski, are a feature characteristic of many psychoneurotic individuals and are seen in some psychoses such as schizophrenia and manic-depressive

---

[15] *Ibid.*, p. 10.

psychosis. Therefore, the symptoms of many "slighter" mental disorders ought to be considered an expression of positive rather than negative compensation and development.

Just as is the case in various developmental crises, such as puberty and sometimes the climacteric, many mental disorders may be the cause as well as the symptom of positive development of the individual, bringing increasing awareness both in retrospection and in prospection, even though there is disadaptation to the present situation. In both former and latter states a psychic complexity arises as a basic factor in the development of a multidimensional structure and in the potential for creativity. Every disease, including mental disease, causes a break in automatic adaptation and often gives impulse to an accelerated development. The stresses of life and the conflict of disadaptation may activate attitudes which until then had no chance of revealing themselves.

The Jacksonian hypothesis that the highest mental levels are most easily injured and are initially involved during illness has not been validated. Pierre Janet's "function of reality" places highest value on synthetic adaptation to the actual situation. However, the majority of outstanding creative minds in the field of art and even of science manifest in great measure an underdevelopment of this function of reality in conditions of everyday life. This indicates that their evolution involves disintegration. In this type of individual a strong instinct of development has overcome a lower "function of reality." Neurasthenics and psychasthenics are in many cases mentally and morally very efficient, though often not able to complete this or that concrete action. Also there is no adequate evidence to support the hypothesis that dissolution begins in higher and newer functions and proceeds downward to simple, automatic ones. The life history of prominent individuals and also of many psychoneurotics reveals a dissolution and even atrophy of simple automatic functions, whereas their higher, complex functions are fully preserved. Gandhi's hunger strike is proof of a complete control of the instinct of self-preservation, and of the instinct of hunger. Many individuals submit consciously to starvation down to a state of inanition out of the sense of duty, or for the sake of love. Others submit consciously to tortures. In many cases of psychoneurosis—for example, obsessional neurosis—we meet with an unimpaired efficiency of the higher functions while the lower functions are weakened, inhibited, or deficient. The recovery of numerous mental patients results in not only their return to their previous state of health but also the attainment of a higher level of mental functioning. Patients often manifest a development of their creative capacities even during the climax of their illness.

Taking into consideration the similarity between certain symptoms of mental diseases, the behavior of highly productive, creative, and intelligent individuals, and the symptoms shown by normal persons during such developmental crises as puberty or the climacteric and during periods of stress, I conclude, contrary to Jackson, that slight morbid symptoms may have a positive influence on the development of most individuals. In like fashion, by examining mental symptoms from the point of view of the development of the personality, I further conclude, unlike Jackson, that positive and negative disintegrative processes in psychopathology can be distinguished.

I find that slighter forms of mental disorder are closely related to an individual's accelerated development, are often indispensable to it, and, indeed, constitute its essential mechanism. This I have termed the process of positive disintegration.

Jackson's practice of labeling a given symptom as morbid cannot be used solely on the analysis of the symptom's structure and pattern. It is necessary to examine its place and significance in the developmental history of a given individual, and its dynamic meaning for him, depending on his age, sex, personality type, and cultural level.

Many symptoms of disintegration are not, as Jackson states, the expression of transition from a complex to a simple level, from a free to an automatic one, or from a hierarchically higher to a lower one, but often just the reverse.

Finally, in partial opposition to and in extension of Jackson's principles of evolution and dissolution, I believe that certain disintegrative processes which appear to injure higher functions in actuality cause the weakening, loosening, and dissolution of primitive structures and lead to evolutionary development of hierarchically higher structures.

8.

Positive Disintegration and Child Development

The period of infancy is a distinctly integrated one since all the activities of an infant are directed to the goal of satisfying the basic necessities. The opposite of integration is disintegration, i.e., structures and dynamisms scattered, separated, split, and not subordinated to a distinct disposing and directing center.

Disintegration is strongly manifested during the developmental periods of childhood. We may observe distinct signs of it in infants, both at about 18 months and at 2½ years of age. Capriciousness, dissipated attention, period of artificiality, animism, and magical thinking are closely connected with a wavering nervous system and unstable psychic structure. During this time a child's moods are changing and its acts are incoherent and very often in contradiction to one another. In the age of opposition, elements of disintegration become stronger.

A later but still typical period of disintegration is the age of puberty, characterized by its lack of emotional balance, its ambivalence, ambitendencies, variation of attitudes either with a feeling of superiority or of inferiority, criticism and self-criticism, often self-dislike, maladaptation to the outer world, and concern with the past or future rather than the present. A lack of psychic balance and disintegration symptoms are also likely to appear in the climacteric period.

HYPEREXCITABILITY

Nervous children, who have increased psychomotor, emotional, imaginative, and sensual or mental psychic excitability and who show strength and perseveration of reactions incommensurate to their stimuli, reveal patterns of disintegration. A child with psychomotor hyperexcitability responds far beyond what is appropriate to the stimuli of his environment, occasioning conflicts within himself and with others. So does the child with increased emotional excitability, whose individual structure contains germs of disintegration (anxiety, phobias, slight states of anguish, and emotional hypersensitivity).

The child with *imaginative* hyperexcitability is not able to agree with his environment; he will often reach out beyond the limits of actual life into a world of dreams and fantasy. He manifests a pronounced maladaptation to reality. The child with *sensory* hyperexcitability, the exaggerated growth of the sensory sphere to the disadvantage of other spheres, may also have difficulties in adapting to his surroundings and in managing himself in conditions demanding reactions of a different kind from sensory ones. The child with *mental* hyperexcitability can also be maladapted, owing to an exaggerated search for explanations and a tendency to intellectualize problems in everyday life.

Psychoneurotic children clearly demonstrate the large field of disintegration and the great variability of its symptoms. Increased excitability here is a minor manifestation, for disorders of thought, of sensation, and of emotional life are more important symptoms. Extreme manifestations of pathological disintegration are psychotic children—most typically schizophrenics.

EMOTIONS

Emotions play a vital role in the psychic life of man. According to Pierre Janet, they have a disintegrating influence upon the mind: "Every emotion acts in a dissolving way upon the mind, diminishes its capacity of synthesis and renders it weaker for a certain time." On the other hand, it is well known that certain feelings, such as love, are elements that mobilize people, particularly children. We often observe a distinct association between increased emotional excitation (nervousness in general) in children and their capabilities. Here we note two contradictory points of view concerning emotions in the psychic life of children: the theory of positive disintegration and Janet's negative view. These two opinions might be reconciled by the acknowledgment of two types of disintegrating action, one of them working positively in the field of a child's development, the other working negatively. Positive disintegration renders the individual's psychic structure especially sensitive to stimuli, causing a deepening and acceleration of his development. Negative disintegration creates disharmony in the child's emotional structure without activation of tendencies to development or to creativity. Thus, in the case of emotional hyperexcitability, a child's susceptibility to exterior and interior stimuli increases, and a positive development of intellectual, moral, and aesthetic values is likely to take place.

INFERIORITY FEELINGS

Similarly, the feeling of self-inferiority, according to Adler's school and to other psychiatrists, may have either a positive or a negative influence upon a child's development, depending on the child's constitutional, intellectual, and moral capacities as well as on the effect of the environment.

The feeling of self-inferiority in children concerns their relationship not only to their surroundings but to themselves. It may be a symptom of multilevel disintegration causing a dispersion and sometimes even a splitting of the child's psychic structure, in which case it leads to the establishment of higher or "better" and lower or "worse" structure in the inner self. Such a process will encourage a growth in judgment, richness of emotional life, and movement toward the formation of a personality. There sometimes also develops a feeling of guilt attached to activities originating at the lower level and to conflicts between lower and higher values in the internal environment of the child.

FRUSTRATION

Frustration is generally considered a negative factor in man's development, but it may also have another aspect. We know of cases in which frustration played a positive role in the lives of individuals endowed with rich moral, intellectual, and aesthetic resources. The examples of Balzac, Fergusson, David, Dryden, and others prove that frustration may lead to positive compensation, may awaken abilities, prompt ambition, increase sensitivity, and contribute to the growth of creativeness and the development of an ideal. Frustration may have a principal part in the self-education of youth for during the period of puberty an attitude of will appears, confirming or rejecting certain values.

PSYCHIC INFANTILISM

Psychic infantilism may also be related to positive development. An individual with this condition may show on the one hand expressions of mental immaturity but on the other hand considerable alertness, an increased psychic sensitiveness, and often very rich intellectual resources. This kind of immaturity in children and young people should not be considered disadvantageous; it is, on the contrary, a potentially positive factor in their development. In many artists, writers, and scientists (for example, Chopin, Slowacki, Shelley, and Veininger) we may observe symptoms of psychic infantilism. The complex of psychic properties which we call infantilism may contain innumerable possibilities of development toward the creative personality.

RECOGNITION OF POSITIVE DISINTEGRATION

The question arises: When may disintegration be considered positive? Examples of positive disintegration may be observed in the psychic phenomena of everyday life. During such periods as the age of opposition, puberty, and maturation we observe the strongest developmental progress, the most intense individual experience, and the greatest transformation of psychic structure.

At the same time, however, we note that the individual undergoes a very serious faltering of equilibrium. Many specialists of this domain in psychiatry consider that these periods partly approach schizophrenia. According to Rorschach, persons of the so-called ambiequal type, who are highly harmonious, are seen mostly in the period of opposition and during the period of puberty, which, as we know, usually are times of disharmony and disintegration. Although some individuals have a disquieting wavering of psychic structure during these periods, they also may begin to display harmonious elements which develop in the course of time. Nervousness and psychic excitability, both characteristic of such a wavering psychic system, are correlated with positive capabilities. Polish, French, and Swiss investigators agree that among capable school children 80 per cent are nervous or show symptoms of slight neurosis.

States of anxiety and of hyperexcitability and certain states of neurosis—self-dislike, depressive reactions, and a feeling of strangeness toward reality, for example—are often connected with the capacity for accelerated development and with psychic subtlety, a delicacy of feeling, and considerable moral development. Most of the mechanisms considered typical of psychoneurosis by Pavlov's school, such as the swaying of balance between the processes of stimulation and inhibition, excessive inhibition or stimulation, and disharmony between activities of the cortex and subcortical centers, or between the first and second signaling system, are phenomena generally observed in sensitive individuals with considerable abilities and potential for a high level of development.

Positive disintegration is also found in the psychopathology of eminent men. Beers, Fergusson, David, Wagner, and Dostoevsky show distinct psychotic or borderline psychotic processes. During or after their illness these men manifested higher forms of creative psychic organization than before. Even when suspecting psychosis, the psychiatrist must refrain from judging the case to be pathological disintegration until the end of the process. The so-called psychopathological symptoms—delusions, anxiety, phobias, depression, feelings of strangeness of oneself, emotional overexcitability, etc.—should not be generally or superficially classified as symptoms of mental disorder and disease since the further development of individuals manifesting them will often prove their positive role in development.

The theory of Jackson and the neo-Jacksonists, who conceive development as the passing from a simple, automatic, well-organized level to a more complicated, less automatic, and not so well-organized level, is based in a certain sense on a one-sided idea of developmental mechanisms, especially as concerns children. First, we may observe well-organized activities on a very high level, and second (contrary to Jackson's theory), disease processes may involve structures of lower or middle levels, not interfering with higher activities. There is no evidence that psychoneuroses are the initial state of every mental disease.

The conception of Freud, stressing the morbidity of conflict between libido and reality, and between the id, ego, and superego, is not a full explanation of the dynamics of normal and pathological development. In my opinion, the conflict within the inner psychic milieu, especially in its multilevel structure, is one of the most important dynamisms in the positive development of personality.

The inner conflict in neurosis, described by Jung as pathological, seems to play a principal role in development, while Pierre Janet's "reality function" plays a synthesizing part in adapting the individual to reality. Janet regards the absence of "reality function" in the inner structure as a cause of psychoneurosis. The theory of positive disintegration implies that the "reality function" undergoes major transformations during development.

It seems probable that certain forms of maladaptation to one's self and to reality, hypersensitivity, lability of psychic structure, and even certain symptoms of internal discord such as self-criticism with a strong emotional accent are elements indispensable in man's development.

During developmental crises and during periods of stress in the lives of children we may find in nervousness, neurosis, and many other disintegration processes hidden germs of positive intellectual and character development. This conclusion is illustrated by a school crisis:

M—, a girl 10 years old of asthenic-schizothymic type, had marked mathematical and scientific abilities and was dutiful, with a tendency to be overly so.

After good progress in one school she was moved to another, more extroverted system, where the teachers were prone to superficial appreciation of their students, basing their opinions on the pupil's boldness and originality.

M—, a rather shy girl with excessive inhibitions, withdrew from these new conditions and for several weeks showed both shyness and anxiety. She obtained marks that were fairly good, but much lower than in her former school. Her anxieties increased; she became resentful, slept badly, lost weight, and was either irritable or withdrawn.

After several months her marks improved, although she lost confidence in some of her teachers. When her parents discussed with her the possibility of moving to another class or another school, she replied: "It seems to me that in another class or school there will be similar teachers. I don't want to change. Always, only some of the teachers and some of the other students will like me. That's the way people are, and that's the way I am." In this case, disintegration occurred in an ambitious girl with a strong sense of justice, resulting in withdrawal and resentment. The fact that she did not wish to transfer to another class or school seems to be explained by emotional exhaustion and, at the same time, an increasingly realistic attitude toward the environment and patterns of interaction with it. This is a sign of partial, still insufficient, but clear rebuilding. Secondary integration is evident in M's new appreciation of herself and others but is still combined with a feeling of disappointment and a certain degree of compromise.

9.

Mental Health as the Progressive Development of Personality

One aspect of the concept of mental health is the relationship of frustration to one's psychic state. A person deprived of the possibility of fulfilling his basic needs experiences frustration. Such deprivation, especially in children and adolescents, often leads to slight or severe psychosomatic disturbances, to various asocial attitudes, e.g., increased egoism, aggressiveness, stealing, and delinquency, or even to psychosis. However, what is the relationship of frustration to mental health when deprivation is deliberately produced by the individual himself? Under these circumstances frustration takes on a different meaning. Individuals with great inner depth, social sensitivity, alterocentrism, and a strong sense of justice may consciously and voluntarily, like Mahatma Gandhi, commit themselves to self-frustration. Such individuals are aware that most people are continually or intermittently deprived of the possibility of realizing their needs. This awareness often constitutes the basis for voluntary acceptance of similar deprivation in the name of social justice. Thus these individuals achieve their goals in personality development. There are, then, two processes of frustration: one involuntary, negative in results; the other conscious and voluntary, often conducive to personality development (in both those who practice it and those for whom it is undertaken).

A similar situation is evident with feelings of inferiority. They may lead to jealousy, anxiety states, depression, or aggressive tendencies. On the other hand, inferiority feelings, the sense of shame and guilt in relation to others and especially toward oneself, may form a basic dynamism for personality development. The sense of inferiority in relation to oneself occurring in a person capable of development is an acknowledgment of having acted incorrectly; there emerges a sense of disharmony between one's own moral possibilities and one's present behavior. Such feelings of inferiority may not be detrimental to the development of the individual but may be a positive element in his development.

It is not within the scope of this chapter either to discuss all the elements which may influence an individual's personality or to isolate any single factor. What should be noted, however, is that any one factor must be considered (so far as total mental health of an individual is concerned) in both time and space. By *space* is meant its position with regard to other factors that may be present; by *time* is meant temporal variability. Therefore, such specific symptoms as anxiety, phobia, or depression may be positive or negative and ought not to be hastily or superficially judged by the psychiatrist.

DIAGNOSIS OF MENTAL HEALTH OR ILLNESS

The psychiatrist should not base his diagnosis of health or illness of a patient exclusively or even primarily on the actual symptoms the patient shows. Symptoms of nervousness in one individual may be automatic, half-conscious, uncreative reactions. In another patient the same symptoms can represent a process of increasing sensitivity, or even remodeling of the personality. Symptoms of unreality and depersonalization can, in one instance, indicate the onset of a psychotic process; in another situation they may signify a process of positive personality development.

Diagnosis of the pathological or healthy nature of the syndromes of inferiority and guilt depends on the role that these syndromes play in the individual, the relation between the individual and the group around him, and whether or not there is an increase in insight and self-awareness. In most cases it is possible to evaluate these factors by an examination of the patient's actual situation. However, in cases of severe neuroses and psychoses the psychiatrist can reach an opinion only after months or even years of observation and investigation which have allowed him to grasp the manifestations of unconscious, genotypic structure and their meaning to the whole personality of the patient.

Actual symptoms of psychoneurosis—or even psychosis—do not tell us much about the fundamental process of the development or the dissolution of an individual. The same symptom picture in two persons may represent very different causal backgrounds and have very different results. The psychiatrist cannot, therefore, prognosticate about a given process on the basis of actual symptoms, any more than he could pronounce a negative and final judgment about a child's personality on the basis of, for example, transient lying, tantrums, opposition, and disobedience. No final prognosis may be based merely on the appearance of any symptom.

Today, the well-known axiom *Mens sana in corpore sano* cannot be taken seriously. There are many physically healthy psychopaths, neurotics, and even psychotics. Conversely, there are many people physically ill whose basic psychic elements function at a high level. In fact, it can be observed that in many individuals physical illness causes changes in psychic structure which lead to increased sensitivity of consciousness, alterocentrism, responsibility, and broader conceptual horizon. Of course, the direction of such phenomena depends, to a large extent, on the specific psychic structure of a particular individual.

Immobility, physical weakness, unpleasant events in the external environment, and changes in the autonomic nervous system often increase the vividness and richness of imagination and deepen one's sensitivity to the external and internal world. Sherrington describes this condition as dissociation between the skeletal muscular function and the functions of thought and speech, while Pavlov describes it in terms of the second signal system typical of psychasthenics. The creative wealth of artists and philosophers is not unrelated to past or current physical ailments. The English poet John Keats, afflicted with tuberculosis wrote, "Such thoughts came seldom when I was healthy." In many creative individuals physical illness accelerates the development of creativity and deepens the personality. From the chaos of symptoms of the physically sick there may emerge elements strengthening talent and developing personality. Surely, whatever meaning we may give to mental health, this is a positive side of it.

DEFINITIONS OF MENTAL HEALTH

In current discussions of mental health a distinction is often made between positive and negative definitions. The negative definition is that mental health is the absence of symptoms of a pathological process or of a pathological constitution. The positive definition invokes the presence of some characteristic such as the fulfillment of one's potentialities, or the ability to love and to work. According to one view, the absence of pathological characteristics is sufficient for a given individual to be regarded as mentally healthy; according to the other, it is necessary to discover positive characteristics in order to consider a person mentally healthy. The first or negative definition is erroneous since psychic symptoms may be signs of positive personality development.

The theory of positive disintegration has it that most states of anxiety, depression, and other symptoms of psychoneurosis are necessary conditions of positive development of the individual. They permit him to become susceptible to factors accelerating and deepening his personality growth. The individual who is nervous or who succumbs to psychoneurotic processes often shows a greater potential for psychic development—psychic health, not illness. Mental health is the progressive development of the personality; therefore, progressive psychic development is the movement toward higher and higher levels of personality functions in the direction of the personality ideal.

The propensity for changing one's internal environment and the ability to influence positively the external environment indicate the capacity of the individual to develop. Almost as a rule, these factors are related to increased mental excitability, depressions, dissatisfaction with oneself, feelings of inferiority and guilt, states of anxiety, inhibitions, and ambivalences—all symptoms which the psychiatrist tends to label psychoneurotic.

Given a definition of mental health as the development of the personality, we can say that all individuals who present active development in the direction of a higher level of personality (including most psychoneurotic patients) are mentally healthy. Also, many psychotic patients (including schizophrenics) who cannot have actual mental health have the potential for it.

The negative formulation of mental health, as we have seen, is static, but easy to describe specifically. The consideration of mental health as progressive development, on the other hand, constitutes a dynamic formulation but is difficult to describe explicitly. One approach would be to list the most frequent characteristics occurring during different stages in the life cycle, but this overemphasizes "average" patterns. Such a formulation becomes more complete, however, by the introduction of exemplary values for these structures.

The question of normality in a person is usually decided on the basis of how similar his personality characteristics are, both in frequency and in force, to those psychosomatic processes most often encountered in a given society. The most frequent and thus "normal" traits express themselves in the following norms: practical rather than theoretical intelligence, predominantly egocentric rather than alterocentric attitudes toward society, and preponderance of the self-preservation, sexual, exploratory, and social instincts. These traits are commonly in compliance with group thinking and behavior and are often accompanied by minor, "safe" dishonesty. Such a group of "normal" traits in a person should, according to many, allow us to describe him as mentally healthy. Can we agree? No. This formulation is humiliating to mankind; a more suitable definition of mental health must contain, besides average values, exemplary ones.

An appraisal of the mental health of an individual must, therefore, be based on the findings of progressive development in the direction of exemplary values. Most psychoneurotics are mentally healthy according to this definition. An individual (even a schizophrenic) who has the ability to develop has potential mental health.

In assessing the mental health of outstanding persons one should apply individual, almost unique, personality norms, for the course of their development must be evaluated in terms of their own personality ideals. These individuals often show accelerated development in one direction or another. They are likely to have psychoneuroses, one-sided skills, little stereotypy in their attitudes, often more or less impaired reality testing, easy transfer of mental tension to the autonomic nervous system, and often outstanding dexterity of higher functions with retardation of lower ones. An accurate evaluation must be based on a thorough knowledge of the history of their life and development.

CREATIVITY AND MENTAL HEALTH

Creativity is the ability for, and realization of, new and original approaches to reality. It is expressed in the new formulation of issues and in original productions arising from unique interrelationships between the psychic internal milieu and the stimuli of the external world. Stereotypy, the automatic repetition of past patterns, is a necessary phase in the development of an individual. It is concerned with activities of everyday life after they have been "learned"—walking, running, eating, and many occupational tasks. Automatic repetitions also occur in mental activities: orderliness in work, systematic functioning, short cuts in calculations, and the everyday association of ideas. The individual who shows personality development always has some stereotypy and some creativity. Stereotypy increases in old people but leads to progressive personality paralysis and mental retardation. The necessity of constantly living in the same cultural milieu with the same people is in a sense stamped with stereotypy. Where curiosity and disquietude do not arise, there is no more than automatic activity. The attitudes of self-criticism, doubt, surprise, and disquietude are essentially healthy and creative.

Creativity is the enemy of stereotypy and automatic activity. A creative person is prospective and inventive even during retrospective contemplation. In the projective method of Rorschach a creative individual will give original answers with kinesthetic perceptions, color sensitivity, many whole responses, and awareness of light and shade. Persons of the ambiequal type, according to Rorschach, are creative individuals.

The ability to take new and original approaches to reality is particularly evident during the developmental stages of life and is often connected in some individuals with periods of emotional crisis, inner conflicts, and difficult life experiences. It seems to demand "turbulence" in the inner environment. The creative attitude commonly accompanies the infantile mental qualities, mental imbalance, and excessive sensitivity found in some adults. Psychoneurotics are very likely to be creative. They often show loosening and disruption of the internal milieu and conflict with the external environment.

Are creative people mentally healthy? A question phrased in this way has to be answered in general in the affirmative. They are not healthy according to the standard of the average individual, but they are healthy according to their unique personality norms and insofar as they show personality development: the acquiring and strengthening of new qualities in the realization of movement toward their personality ideal.

MENTAL HEALTH AND THE PERSONALITY IDEAL

Mental health is accompanied by some degree of ability to transform one's psychological type in the direction of attaining one's ideal. During the course of development, an individual experiences self-criticism and feelings of inferiority toward himself. The third factor (which has been discussed previously) becomes mobilized. In building his character an individual often recognizes tendencies which he cannot reconcile with the need to develop traits other than those he already has. For example, he may aim at transforming his excessively schizothymic and introverted attitude by developing syntony, alterocentrism, and the ability to live with others.

If the individual possesses opposite mental characteristics, he may aim to go beyond a narrow extroversion through reflection, meditation, and the developed ability to remain in solitude. These changes may be necessary to complete and cultivate his present structure in the realization of his personality ideal. During the changes he experiences the processes of positive disintegration, through which his psychological type becomes more complex and is supplemented with new, and to some degree opposite, characteristics. This leads to development of his inner psychic environment, a deepening and enlargement of his life experience, and, gradually, secondary integration. The transformation of psychological type, the deepening and broadening of personality, is directly related to symptoms of positive disintegration. Mental health thus necessarily involves some psychological symptoms.

EFFICIENCY OF MENTAL FUNCTIONS

The efficiency of basic mental functions is too often given as the prime characteristic of an individual's mental health. However, even granting that we could agree on what these functions are, insurmountable difficulties exist in formulating a definition of mental health. The efficiency of basic mental functions increases and diminishes depending on the time of day or night, overwork, and motivation, as well as on the sense of well-being, the developmental stage of life, physical health, and many other factors. We cannot, therefore, regard simple inefficiency as signifying mental pathology. Moreover, some people show signs of incompetence in one area but marked efficiency in another area, on a different level and of a different scope. This observation applies particularly to psychoneurotic individuals, who often have great inner depth. Efficiency will be different in the asthenic-schizothymic, in psychocyclic, introverted, and extroverted types, and in people with increased psychic excitability. Also, during the course of development, efficiency of lower functions will be lower during periods of positive disintegration than it has been previously. However, efficiency of higher functions may be increased. Efficiency of a primitive kind thus gradually weakens, giving place to a growing efficiency on a higher level. In order to decide whether a given instance of inefficiency is healthy or pathological, a multidimensional approach is necessary.

THE CONCEPT OF ADAPTATION

In many psychiatric textbooks the ability to adapt to changing conditions of life is given as one of the characteristics of mental health. What is meant by this concept of adaptation? Does it mean clearly understanding various types of environmental reality and various human personality patterns, including their level of development, and on this knowledge basing appropriate behavior in accordance with one's principles? Or does it mean greater or lesser resignation of one's own point of view, principles, and modes of behavior for the sake of resolution of conflict?

The first formulation is in accordance with the demands of mental health; the second is not. The developing individual should understand reality as completely as possible. He should not react too emotionally to the difficulties emerging from it. He may even wisely involve himself in resistances, conflicts, and the consequent life difficulties where an unavoidable situation demands nonadaptation if he is to be consistent with his moral and social points of view. Such an attitude practiced consistently contributes to the formation of moral individuality.

THE MULTIDIMENSIONAL VIEW

Experience, reflection, and the endeavor to reach a higher level of personality make a human being human. The poet Keats noted that it is impossible for man to develop without his sorrows as well as his joys. Sadness, depression, discontent with oneself, shame, guilt, and inferiority are essential for development, as are also the experience of feelings of joy and creativity. The sense of well-being may characterize a person who is developing, but it may also be present in some syndromes such as hypomania or accompany severe organic pathology such as general paresis and Korsakoff's syndrome. Moreover, the sense of mental ill health may often accompany the processes of accelerated personality development.

Herbert Spencer said that he would prefer to be a dissatisfied Socrates than a satisfied animal. We know that at certain stages of intensive psychic development (puberty, for example) negative moods predominate. Of course, a permanent, an unchanging mood of depression is not creative, but states of hypomania or depression, euphoria or sadness, are characteristic of certain phases of creativity.

A tendency to make global syntheses characterizes creative individuals at the height of their creativity. This is usually followed by a phase of self-criticism and distrust in one's creativity. And here again an accurate assessment of whether we are dealing with a healthy or a pathological process is not possible without a multidimensional temporospatial formulation of the individual's internal environment.

In states of psychoneurosis and in frustration a negative feeling state predominates; yet in most of these states we find creative dynamic processes. Kierkegaard's "fear and trembling" is an apt example, as are the creative developmental elements in the neurotic symptoms of Proust, Keats, and David.

SELF-EDUCATION AND AUTOPSYCHOTHERAPY

The capacity to educate himself depends on the existence in an individual of the "object-subject" process, the ability to experience dissatisfaction with himself, and a sense of shame, guilt, and inferiority. The basic condition for self-education is the possession of a high level of self-awareness, namely, the ability to recognize the state of one's internal environment. This contributes to the development of self-control and self-approval, which are further elements in the process of self-education. The process of self-education also assumes the presence of a clear and dynamic personality ideal.

An individual capable of developing may be characterized by various forms of increased excitability or nervousness, and even by psychoneurosis. Mental tension, internal and external conflicts—indeed the whole process of disintegration—cause a sense of ill health. Nevertheless, such an individual possesses a sense of his own creativity, an awareness of the transformation of his character, and a knowledge of his personality ideal. These contribute to his ability to effect autopsychotherapy. Realization of the complexities of both the internal and the external environment and of one's own hierarchy of values enables one to reach a higher level of integration through autopsychotherapy, not merely to return to the previous state (*restitutio in integrun*). An individual possessing these qualities usually has a great deal of knowledge about himself, his conflicts, and their role in compensation and sublimation. His clear personality ideal allows him to determine the direction of the secondary integration.

It is not internal conflict, nervousness, or even neurosis which signifies mental disease. These symptoms, side by side with the capacity for autopsychotherapy and its participation in reaching a higher developmental level, indicate that the individual is mentally healthy. Psychic symptoms within one's structure and dynamic processes do not mean mental illness. True disturbance of mental health exists only in cases of negative disintegration. As has been made plain, syndromes of nervousness or psychoneurosis (and sometimes psychosis) may indicate not mental illness but rather developmental possibilities and unfolding mental health. In "pathological" cases of this kind the individual can determine his own fate and transformation. Such autopsychotherapy is nothing but self-education under especially difficult conditions.

PRIMARY INTEGRATION

The state of primary integration is a state contrary to mental health. A fairly high degree of primary integration is present in the average person; a very high degree of primary integration is present in the psychopath. The more cohesive the structure of primary integration, the less the possibility of development; the greater the strength of automatic functioning, stereotypy, and habitual activity, the lower the level of mental health. The psychopath is only slightly, if at all, capable of development; he is deaf and blind to stimuli except those pertaining to his impulse-ridden structure, to which intelligence is subordinated. The absence of the development of personality means the absence of mental health.

MENTAL HEALTH AND POSITIVE DISINTEGRATION

During the stages of opposition and puberty, during breakdowns, depressions, and creative upsurges which violate the stabilized psychic structure, the psychiatrist may observe psychic disintegration, development of "new things," decrease in automatic behavior, nonadjustment to the environment, and an increase in self-awareness, self-control, and psychic development. In these periods the individual develops an attitude of dissatisfaction with himself and a sense of shame, guilt, and inferiority. Also, the capacity for prospection and retrospection expands, the activity of the third factor increases, and there is a sense of reality of the personality ideal and the need to achieve it.

What is new, higher, richer, must in a large measure grow from the loosening and disruption of what is old, simple, poorer, integrated, and nondynamic. Achievement of the "new," the "higher," is almost always connected with a process which over a period of time must demonstrate a stronger or weaker, narrow or wide process of disintegration. Therefore, the stages of disintegration are related to creativity, general psychic development, growth of self-awareness, and mental health.

During the stage of opposition in the small child, during the stage of puberty, in states of nervousness and psychoneurosis, and under conditions of internal conflict, disharmony, and dysfunction in one's own internal environment, the third factor arises and becomes more or less pronounced. Self-awareness, self-approval, and self-disapproval play a basic role in the development of the third factor. It relates negatively and positively, and therefore selectively, to specific aspects of the external environment. This third factor always appears during periods of positive disintegration and is connected with creative, dynamic processes in prospective and retrospective attitudes and with purposeful nonadaptation. It is a basic factor for the realization of one's personality ideal. It is the primary dynamic element in the development of dissatisfaction with oneself, shame, guilt, and inferiority and in the building of one's own hierarchical internal environment. The development of personality, and consequently mental health, is clearly related to the activities of the third factor.

The process of mental disintegration in an individual leads to symptoms of multilevel disintegration. This results in disruption within the internal environment, in the rise of a sense of "object-subject," in the growth of an awareness of higher and lower levels in the hierarchy of one's values, and in the development of an attitude of prospection and retrospection. All these contribute to the movement of the disposing and directing center to a higher level, to the emergence of the third factor, and to the development of a personality ideal. The activity of the third factor enables the individual to see more clearly his personal ideal, which, as it becomes more distinct, has greater influence on the development of the personality. Under these conditions the individual becomes more cohesive in the area of his values and more socially sensitive and alterocentric, at the same time retaining his unique individual qualities. This situation leads to a high level of mental health.

Everyday experience and experiments of developmental psychology indicate that one-sided specialization narrows personality development. Yet specialization (as long as it is temporary or relates only to a limited range of activities) is necessary and useful in modern society. Creativity, on the other hand, is almost always allied to a broad intellectual sensitivity and to a multidimensional attitude. The developing individual cannot submit to narrow specialization except at the cost of a loss in creativity.

The increasing development of technology has become a basic element in our civilization. Technology is essential for the progress of modern society and has provided man with mass production, efficient and widespread distribution of goods and services, and thus a considerable degree of material well-being. Traditional humanism emphasizes a broader educational background, moral and social values, and the uniqueness of the individual. Both components are necessary for the development of individuals and society, but the humanistic orientation must play a dominant role in relation to technology. The reverse relationship would weaken the psychic development of the individual and consequently diminish the potentials of society. Technology increases rather than minimizes the potentiality for both individual and group psychopathology.

The concept of mental health must be based on a multidimensional view of personality development. Higher levels of personality are gradually reached both through adaptation to exemplary values and through disadaptation to lower levels of the external and internal environments. Development proceeds through the transformation of one's type, the widening of one's interests and capabilities, and the gradual approach toward one's personality ideal through the process of positive disintegration and the activity of the third factor. Thus development moves—in partial accordance with Jackson's formulation—from what is simple to what is complex, and from what is automatic to what is spontaneous. Mental health is the development of personality toward a more elevated hierarchy of goals set by the personality ideal. In this definition, mental health means the continual striving toward further personality development.

Index

Publisher's Catalogue

The Prosperous Series

#1 The Prosperous Coach: Increase Income and Impact for You and Your Clients (Steve Chandler and Rich Litvin)

#2 The Prosperous Hip Hop Producer: My Beat-Making Journey from My Grandma's Patio to a Six-Figure Business (Curtiss King)

* * *

Devon Bandison

Fatherhood Is Leadership: Your Playbook for Success, Self-Leadership, and a Richer Life

Sir Fairfax L. Cartwright

The Mystic Rose from the Garden of the King

Steve Chandler

37 Ways to BOOST Your Coaching Practice: PLUS: the 17 Lies That Hold Coaches Back and the Truth That Sets Them Free

50 Ways to Create Great Relationships

Business Coaching (Steve Chandler and Sam Beckford)

Crazy Good: A Book of CHOICES

Death Wish: The Path through Addiction to a Glorious Life

Fearless: Creating the Courage to Change the Things You Can

RIGHT NOW: Mastering the Beauty of the Present Moment

The Prosperous Coach: Increase Income and Impact for You and Your Clients (The Prosperous Series #1) (Steve Chandler and Rich Litvin)

Shift Your Mind, Shift the World: Revised Edition

Time Warrior: How to defeat procrastination, people-pleasing, self-doubt, over-commitment, broken promises and chaos

Wealth Warrior: The Personal Prosperity Revolution

Kazimierz Dąbrowski

Positive Disintegration

The Philosophy of Essence: A Developmental Philosophy Based on the Theory of Positive Disintegration

Charles Dickens

A Christmas Carol: A Special Full-Color, Fully-Illustrated Edition

James F. Gesualdi

Excellence Beyond Compliance: Enhancing Animal Welfare Through the Constructive Use of the Animal Welfare Act

Janice Goldman

Let's Talk About Money: The Girlfriends' Guide to Protecting Her ASSets

Sylvia Hall

This Is Real Life: Love Notes to Wake You Up

Christy Harden

Guided by Your Own Stars: Connect with the Inner Voice and Discover Your Dreams

I Heart Raw: Reconnection and Rejuvenation Through the Transformative Power of Raw Foods

Curtiss King

The Prosperous Hip Hop Producer: My Beat-Making Journey from My Grandma's Patio to a Six-Figure Business (The Prosperous Series #2)

David Lindsay

A Blade for Sale: The Adventures of Monsieur de Mailly

Abraham H. Maslow

The Psychology of Science: A Reconnaissance

Being Abraham Maslow (DVD)

Maslow and Self-Actualization (DVD)

Albert Schweitzer

Reverence for Life: The Words of Albert Schweitzer

William Tillier

Personality Development Through Positive Disintegration: The Work of Kazimierz Dąbrowski

Margery Williams

The Velveteen Rabbit: or How Toys Become Real

Colin Wilson

New Pathways in Psychology: Maslow and the Post-Freudian Revolution

Join our Mailing List:
www.MauriceBassett.com

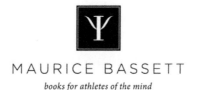

MAURICE BASSETT
books for athletes of the mind

Lightning Source UK Ltd.
Milton Keynes UK
UKHW021808010319
338299UK00014B/279/P